Birds,
Beasts & *Bature*

Birds, Beasts & *Bature*

VIC SMITH

The Pentland Press
Edinburgh – Cambridge – Durham – USA

First published in 1996 by
The Pentland Press Ltd
1 Hutton Close,
South Church
Bishop Auckland
Durham

ISBN 1-85821-404-1

Typeset by Carnegie Publishing, 18 Maynard St, Preston
Printed and bound by Antony Rowe Ltd, Chippenham

For June

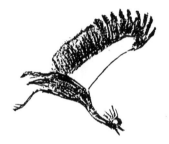

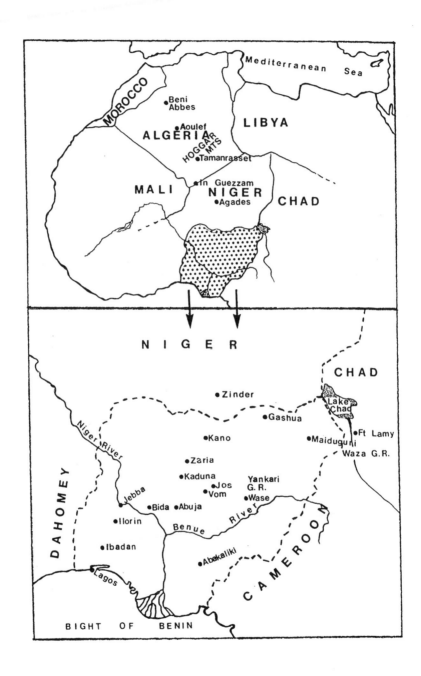

Contents

Illustrations

Birds, Beasts & *Bature*

Acknowledgements

I AM INDEBTED TO JEAN AND IAN TAYLOR AND TONY THORNE for scrutinising earlier drafts of the manuscript and for making so many helpful suggestions; to Dennis Walker for advising me on the few phrases of Hausa I have included; to the companionship of so many colleagues and friends who contributed to making my brief ten years in Nigeria such a memorable experience.

Foreword

MANY TIMES EACH WEEK I WOULD HAVE HEARD *sannu bature* (pronounced 'Batoury'), the polite greeting used by the Hausa of Northern Nigeria when addressing expatriate people of European descent, especially those from Britain.

During that interesting and exciting period before and after Nigeria gained Independence in 1960, I had the opportunity to combine my work as a veterinary research officer studying animal diseases in that country, with my lifelong interest studying birds and animals in a country where there was still so much to learn about the native fauna.

In the process of assimilating a lot of knowledge and dispensing crumbs of advice, I was also rewarded with little glimpses into the lives, customs, habits and behaviour of some Nigerians I met. It was generally a happy time and a period in my life of which I still have the fondest memories.

Born in India, educated in Britain and resident in Australia from the time I left Nigeria in 1966, I look back on my years in West Africa as a rewarding experience. How fortunate I was to witness the transition of a former British Protectorate into a Republic within the Commonwealth.

Thirty years may seem a long time to remember accurately episodes in one's life, but my memories of events have been constantly reinforced by films and photographs, by diaries and letters and by several articles on the Nigerian birdlife which I wrote during that period.

GOODE BEACH, WESTERN AUSTRALIA, 1995.

Introduction

VICTOR, you must look at THIS!'

My mum always called me Victor when I was tiny, to distinguish me from Vic, my father, for we shared the same initials. He had been born in the year of Queen Victoria's Golden Jubilee and I was named after him with a singular lack of originality.

Aged about four, I was reluctant to open my eyes in the intense glare of the Indian sun, while recovering from what I was told much later was a common eye affliction, *Contagious Ophthalmia*, which had responded to copious bathing with boracic eyewashes but left me intensely photophobic.

I must have prised an eye open and through a flood of tears I recall seeing a bundle of leaves in the creeper growing up the verandah of our flat-roofed bungalow in Delhi.

'. . . THIS!' turned out to be the exquisite nest of a tailor bird, leaves sewn together and the pocket filled with a soft lining of kapok. In the nest were two eggs. In Kipling's story of the mongoose 'Rikki-Tikki-Tavi,' a bedtime story I knew well, Darzee the tailor bird played an important part.

From a nearby window I was allowed to watch the young nestlings reared and as a result my eyesight was soon restored to normal. This early childhood experience sowed in me the seeds of an interest and fascination in birds which has persisted all through my life. This interest was later fostered at boarding preparatory school in England and later still in the Scottish Borders where my father retired after serving thirty years in India as a Banker.

Our relationship was almost like grandfather-grandson, for when he retired at the age of just over fifty, the year before war broke out, I was only twelve, with no brothers or sisters. It was as if he was eager to make up for the enforced separations between us that his long tours in India had entailed. After I had been placed in a boarding preparatory school at the tender age of six, he returned to India for his last tour and did not see me for nearly five years.

My father was of the old 'Hunting, Fishing and Shooting' tradition and once he had retired he lavished on me some of the pleasures he had enjoyed during his childhood. Shooting for the pot with a little 20-bore shotgun I was entrusted with from my early teens, not only made me a provider during those lean war years, when father was busy commanding the local 'Dad's Army' in the little town of Moffat just north of the Scottish border. It also encouraged in me a deep appreciation of a countryside full of animal and bird life. Even if the bag was nil, I could still pit my skills against vermin, wily wood-pigeons or carrion crows. How much I used to enjoy just sitting by riverside or amongst the heather, in old soberly-coloured clothing, just watching what went on around me. Constantly carried by me during those days were father's old binoculars, the same pair he had worn when he was awarded a Military Cross at Cambrai in 1917.

A keen horseman himself, father always seemed to regret that in those austere wartime years he was unable to provide me with the opportunities for riding which he had enjoyed as a youngster and later out in India where polo, pig-sticking, point-to-point paperchases and some racing as a gentleman-rider had been so much a part of his life. During the Great War he had served with distinction in France and Palestine with an Indian Cavalry Regiment, part of the time in the Second Bengal Lancers, I was delighted to tell my school mates later.

Horses made me apprehensive, yet even from those early days on that same Delhi verandah, where two cocker spaniels, Biddy and Lassie, between them seemed to produce an astonishing number of pups, there were always dogs, and later cats, in our household. I assume my love for animals and a desire to be able to do something for them stemmed from those early days.

I spent the war years studying for entrance into a veterinary college, at Giggleswick Public School (nowadays referred to as an Independent School) set in the rugged limestone country of the West Riding of Yorkshire. My studies were interrupted during the last year of the War when the R.A.F. had no further use for my services in their Volunteer Reserve, the RAFVR, and at short notice, just after my eighteenth birthday, I was conscripted into the Army, with no chance of more deferment. I missed seeing any active service because the war finished before my training was completed, but I served in India up to the time of Partition and later in Hong Kong.

Exercises near the Khyber Pass and Internal Security diversions around the Indian-Pakistan border made life interesting as a signaller and Fusilier in a distinguished Irish regiment. I was even enticed, but refused, the offer of a short-term commission if I signed on, but my time in the Army seemed a complete waste of time, a thumb-twiddling exercise, learning all the dodges of the old soldier. Yet the delays were very necessary because many service personnel with much longer service than my meagre three years were also awaiting university entrance.

In 1948, aged 22, I eventually started the five year course at the Royal (Dick) Veterinary College in Edinburgh as a first year student.

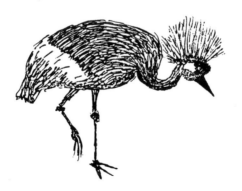

The crowned Crane

CHAPTER I

1957 – First Impressions of Nigeria

LATE IN 1956 an advertisement in *The Veterinary Record*, the journal of the British Veterinary Association, attracted my attention. Veterinary Research Officers were required in Nigeria, one of the British Protectorates on the West Coast of Africa, at the Federal Department of Veterinary Research Laboratories in Vom on the central plateau. In most atlases of that period, British Colonies and Protectorates were the countries shown in pink. When I looked it up, there on the map of Africa was Nigeria, the fourth pink country from the left.

The advertisement described pleasant working conditions at an altitude of 4,000 feet more or less in the centre of Nigeria, where the climate was healthy. Generous leave in Britain was granted every eighteen months. Somewhere else I had read '*The Plateau of Nigeria is an ornithologist's paradise*'.

I had qualified as a veterinary surgeon and became a Member of the Royal College of Veterinary Surgeons in 1953. My initial euphoria palled some three years later when, while working as an assistant in general practice in the Midlands of England, I was laid low with Brucellosis, the consequences of which made me wonder whether general practice was right for me.

Needing a change of direction in my work and relishing an opportunity to look at birds different from those I knew in Britain, I was prompted to give Nigeria a go, in spite of my father advising me against applying. He reminded me that Nigeria was due to get its independence in three years so long-term prospects would be poor. Also he was sure the climate would be unhealthy, though I suspect he was thinking of Nigeria as still having the reputation of being *The White Man's Grave*.

After an interview at the Colonial Office in London, I was accepted though not without a little argument. On the interview board a former Director from Vom, Marshall, pointed out my complete lack of experience in matters tropical, to which I mumbled a retort that given the chance I would gain that experience. Needless to say the first formal offer from the Colonial Office firmly suggested that I would be better off as a Veterinary Officer in the field in Northern Nigeria.

My heart already set on the *'ornithologist's paradise'* bit, I turned the offer down. Fortunately the Director in Vom, Dr Ian Taylor, responded to my rather plaintive cable to him and rapidly had the offer changed. In subsequent correspondence from him and others in Nigeria who kindly wrote to me, I received a lot of useful and practical advice. This was supplemented by a week-long course called LIVING ABROAD, sponsored by the Colonial Office for the benefit of new recruits, on which I learnt that items of clothing like topis and spinepads, still listed in Griffiths McAllister's catalogue, were not really necessary. I also learnt that the Crown Agents for the Colonies, who looked after administrative matters, were always addressed 'Gentlemen, . . .' and that one always signed in what I thought was a most archaic and humiliating fashion, '. . . I have the honour to be, Gentlemen, your humble and obedient servant.'

West Africa was serviced by Elder Dempster Lines, which provided a thirteen day cruise out of Liverpool to Lagos, calling at other West African ports on the way. Not long after appointment, I travelled out on their flagship, M. V. *Aureol,* leaving my wife and son in Britain to join me later. By March 1957 I found myself in Vom, accompanied by Lassie, a sort of labrador-cross, whom I had taken out with me by sea. As I stepped off the train at Bukuru, the nearest station to Vom, before dawn after a two day journey up country from Lagos, I was pleasantly surprised to find all my nineteen crates on the ground beside me. Bukuru did not even boast a platform.

The Catering Rest House in Vom, an admirable institution only a stone's throw from the laboratory buildings, consisted of self-contained chalets with a central dining-room. I was accommodated there for a few days until a house could be found for me. By the time my wife, June, and son Roger, then three months old, joined me a month later, I was already installed temporarily in a house whose regular occupants were away on leave.

Arriving at the end of the dry season, I was a bit disillusioned by the dust, the intense dryness of the air and hardly a bird in sight. It felt strange to be transported from verdant Britain into this barren landscape, which I was seeing at the worst time of year, but no doubt June found the transition even more marked having flown out.

Vom was out at the end of a sealed road, sixteen miles south-west of Jos, the Provincial capital, which was also our nearest shopping centre. The local airport was a couple of miles south of Jos. Apart from a large Mission Hospital a few miles further south, Vom was made up more or less entirely of the Veterinary Research Laboratory buildings, a school for training veterinary assistants and houses for Senior and Junior staff. Adjacent were a Research establishment for studying Trypanosomiasis (animal diseases related to the dreaded Sleeping Sickness of humans), a Mission School and a Dairy, which collected milk from the Fulani cattlemen and turned it into butter, cheese and skim milk powder.

The Plateau of Nigeria was occupied by white men early in the century, when small military expeditions first reached the southern end near Pankshin. Prospectors later penetrated further and found alluvial tin; that together with the good grazing and the healthier climate had encouraged the first tin-mining companies to move in.

Prior to this invasion the Plateau was populated solely by several pagan (non-Moslem) tribes, all at war with each other, and all considered fair game by the marauding Arab or Moslem slavers. It was customary for local agents to collect these pagan slaves, many of whom were exported across the desert or to the northern towns of Nigeria. Some of the rocky outcrops around Vom still showed signs of primitive rock barriers supposedly erected by the pagans in the past for defence.

Around Vom the local tribe was the Birom. Their clusters of grass huts, thatched with grass and surrounded by dense cactus-like fences (really a species of *Euphorbia),* were to be found all around Vom. Adjacent to each family group, crops were cultivated during the wet season, small plots of yams, guinea corn, bullrush millet and the grass-like *Acha,* from which they brewed a potent beer. Some women still wore bunches of leaves fore and aft, the length of the stalk indicating which tribe they hailed from.

The Birom were relatively friendly to outsiders and the first Christian Mission Hospital on the Plateau was founded in 1922 at Vwang, known in later years as Vom Mission Hospital. The legendary Dr Percy Barnden retired in 1958 after 36 years of devoted service to the tribes of the Plateau. He was an astonishing person, possessing degrees in medicine, theology and engineering. Not only a dedicated medical missionary, abolishing such heathen practices as Trial-by-Ordeal and treating major tropical diseases like leprosy, tuberculosis, yaws, elephantiasis and river blindness, he applied his engineering skills to maintaining roads and designing and constructing bridges. Near Vom two suspension bridges designed by him were called Barnden Bridges. One of them, which spanned a considerable gorge near Miango to the west of Vom, was not for the faint-hearted. These bridges were designed to carry vehicles, provided your car was narrow enough to pass through the stone arches

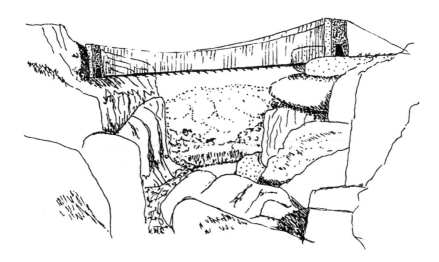

Barnden Bridge at Miango

at either end, but not the much heavier lorries which plied many of the bush roads.

Soon after settling into our first house, we acquired a steward, a young mission-trained Birom called Dantiyi whom we retained for the whole time we were in Nigeria, upgrading him to cook-steward later. Though there was at first considerable room for improvement with his cooking skills, he learnt willingly and was honest. In addition to several of the local dialects, he spoke reasonable English though not without some confusion to start with. When he sorted out the washing, June's bras somehow became "Knickers-for-up"!

All household staff were instructed to boil and filter drinking water and store it in old liquor bottles in the refrigerator. This on occasion could lead to confusion, as at one memorable drink's party, when a Dutchman, Harm Brandsma, expecting his usual gin, exclaimed loudly, 'This is bludy water!' As Roger became older he was trained only to drink water from the refrigerator.

In fact Vom water supply was excellent, yet this regular routine of boiling and filtering ensured that in the bush, perhaps using dirty water drawn from a well, this simple health precaution would be automatically observed. Our daily milk, collected from the farm in a large saucepan, was pasteurised in much the same way by just bringing to the boil. When allowed to cool, the thick clotted cream, like the finest Devonshire product, was skimmed off and the rest of the milk was bottled and stored in the refrigerator.

The choice of house staff was entirely a personal one, and there were plenty to choose from. Vulgar comparisons were made between the suitability of various tribal members for service in the household. Hausa were reputed to be all *Dirt-and-Dignity*. Those from the south, particularly Ibo, were supposedly all *Swank-and-Sweat*. We found these comparisons unfair, for my many colleagues and friends with either Hausa or Ibo servants thought highly of them.

9

Vom, a small area of Federal Territory in the Northern Region of Nigeria, was in the domain of the Moslem Hausa people. Many expatriates eager to learn to speak Hausa found it best to have Hausa servants. In fact had I gone out to Nigeria as a Veterinary Officer in the Northern Region I would have been banished to the bush for three months or so with a retinue of Hausa staff and been compelled to learn their language, not a difficult one to learn under such circumstances.

Most expatriates in Vom tried to learn Hausa, in fact I took lessons under the guidance of Mallam Yahaya Lottu, the despatch clerk in the Laboratory. I regretted not learning their language better, but I was handicapped slightly by my early years in India where I picked up a smattering of childish Hindustani or Urdu, and later a sort of barrack-room lingo during my two years in India prior to partition of that subcontinent. I tended to remember some words in Hausa, some in Urdu, thus spoke a sort of bastardised Esperanto.

Hausa were very polite people, but had a keen eye for caricature, reflected in the nicknames they gave most expatriates. Many had two nicknames, though one was a very private one and never divulged. I never learnt mine, but one of my colleagues was known as *Agwagwa* – 'He that walks like a duck,' another *Ungulu*, because of his vulture-like stoop, and another as *Bunsuru*, because his chin stuck out like a billy goat. By way of retaliation, some Nigerians were graced with nicknames mimicking their real names, which sounded like 'Black-&-Decker,' 'Festering Sam,' or 'Bellyache.'

The customary titles of the Hausa were 'Mallam' (literally Teacher or Mister) and 'Alhaji' for those who had performed the *Haj*, the pilgrimage to Mecca. Greetings, a sort of litany and response, formed an important part of their opening chit-chat. One soon got accustomed to the inevitable *Sannu Bature* and other phrases such as *Rankai dade* ('May you live long') and *Barka da aiki* ('Greetings at your work', whether working or not!).

Some phrases were soon learnt and readily dropped in the conversation, like, *Ina zuwa* ('I am coming'), *Na gode, dyawa* ('Thank you very much'), *Lafiya lau* ('I am well') and *Hankali* ('Slowly'). A favourite expression,

Ba kome shi ke nan seemed to be the equivalent of 'She'll be right' in the Australian vernacular.

Some words readily became anglicised. The words 'Dash' (the back-hander, greasing the palm) was derived from *Haraji*. The acronym BG, from *Bayan gida* (literally 'Behind the house') meant the thunderbox or dunny in the days when it was a separate convenience, but BG was still used to refer to the toilet, though houses in Vom all had 'mod. Cons.'.

In the Laboratory, however, English was the language of necessity. Errors in giving instructions in local dialects could, and indeed did sometimes have disastrous results. Being a Federal organisation, there were staff from all regions. One had to speak precisely and not use slang or colloquialisms. I recall being told of a perfectly true incident which occurred in the veterinary clinic in Jos just prior to my arrival. The veterinary officer told his veterinary assistant to give a valuable pedigree dog, recently imported at great cost, its rabies shot, meaning vaccine, while he chatted with the owner in the clinic. The veterinary assistant got it all wrong, took the dog through to the back and the next moment there was a very final 'Bang' from outside.

More important instructions were best written and acknowledged in writing. A bellow for 'Messenger' would bring a khaki-uniformed figure, clutching not a cleft stick as I had first anticipated, but a small Despatch Book in which one wrote the nature of the message, be it a note or a file, which the recipient signed to acknowledge receipt.

Telephones worked through an old PBX exchange and had to be hand-cranked to arouse the operator and again cranked to ring off at the end of the conversation. During a long conversation with numerous pauses for thought, the operator was inclined to interrupt in a sing-song voice, 'Finished, please? – Finished? – Finished?' and one had to be alert to avoid being cut off.

I soon learnt that Nigeria had a pastoral economy which revolved around the successful harvesting of cash crops and the well-being of the livestock, most of the cattle, sheep and goats being owned by the nomadic Fulani tribes.

Strangely the nomadic nature of the indigenous cattle led to relatively efficient methods of disease control. The Fulani cattlemen owned small herds which represented their entire wealth and they migrated twice a year in search of green pastures for their cattle. At the onset of the dry season they moved down to the larger rivers where the flood basins or *Fadamas* provided ample grazing. The movement was the other way,

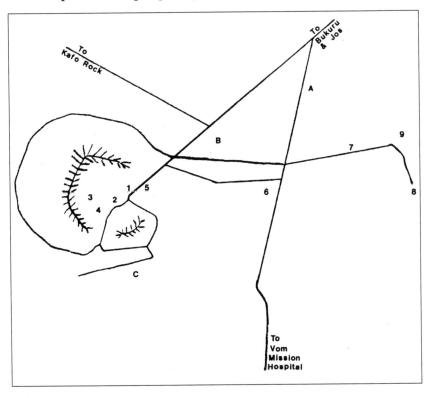

A. Plateau Dairy (Nigerian Creameries). B. St. Joseph's Catholic Mission School.
C. W.A. Institute for Trypanosomiasis Research (later N.I.T.R.).

1. *Administration and New Laboratory.*	2, 3.	*Old Laboratory buildings.*
4. Vom Catering Rest House.	5.	Veterinary school and clinic.
6. Vom Village.	7.	E.P.U.
8. L.I.C.	9.	D.V.R.'s house.

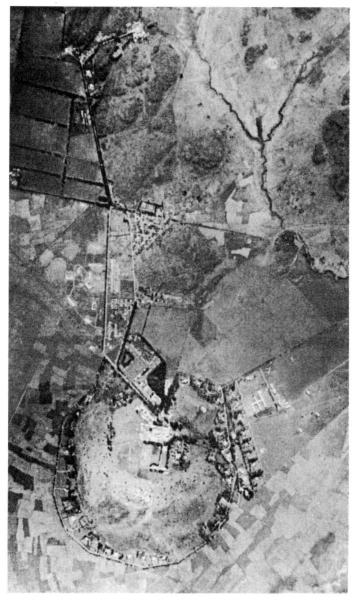

The Federal Department of Veterinary Research, VOM, from the air, about 1964. North is at the top.

when the wet season started, and many herds appeared on the Plateau where the pastures were lush and grass grew shoulder high.

Control posts manned by veterinary assistants were positioned on the main cattle migration routes and as the cattle passed through they received their free vaccinations and treatment. It was far more practical to prevent the many diseases by vaccination than attempt to treat sick animals. Cattle tax was sometimes levied on the Fulani as they passed through the control posts so some cattle owners were known to by-pass such places, otherwise the vaccine coverage was generally good. It was one of our jobs in Vom to produce the vaccines.

The Laboratories at Vom were first started in the early 1920s on the site already chosen some ten years previously as the Veterinary Headquarters for Nigeria. Such a central place was thought to be eminently suitable for controlling the Chief Veterinary Officers in their regions, but one of the earlier Nigerian Governors, in his annual report to the Colonial Secretary, was so irritated by the site that he referred to Vom as 'The Veterinary Headquarters shut away in the remote and rocky fastness of the High Plateau.'

Early colonial veterinary administrators certainly had an eye for selecting attractive, indeed isolated localities, usually sited at a high altitude where the climate was healthier. The precedents were set at Onderstepoort in South Africa, Kabete in Kenya and Mukteswar, like a monastery at the end of an interminably-long mountain road in the Himalayan foothills.

The first task of those veterinary laboratories, in the early years of the colonial era, was to produce Rinderpest antiserum, and later vaccines, for this fatal cattle disease, which was at that time prevalent through much of Africa and Asia.

The site of the Laboratory at Vom, selected by F. Brandt in 1922, was within the weathered cone of an extinct volcano about half a mile in diameter. By 1957, when I arrived, the place had grown enormously. A simple network of roads around the station all bore the names of former Directors or of pioneers in veterinary science and administration who had worked many years in the past in Vom. I suppose I fancifully wondered whether my name would ever be honoured. We first lived in Kearney Crescent and later moved to a house in Henderson Drive, but I recall a Mettam Court and a Simmonds Way. Also remembered were Brandt, Beaton and Marshall.

Senior professional and technical staff were accommodated in houses on the perimeter of the cone, all facing outwards along Henderson Drive. A definite distinction of class existed. All professional or technical staff, which included all the expatriates and few Nigerians when I first arrived, were in the Senior Service, whereas the rest of the Nigerian workforce were in the Junior Service. Even within the Senior Service there had been a distinct observation of rank, which was only just being broken down when I arrived. For instance, socializing between professional and technical staff had been actively discouraged and even the use of first names in the work arena was frowned upon. This attitude, I am glad to say, changed radically during the lead-up to Nigerian independence.

The Laboratory poultry farm, called rather grandly The Egg Production Unit (EPU), provided fertile eggs for the manufacture of some of the viral vaccines. It was situated along the road to the farm, known as the Livestock Investigation Centre (LIC), which, in addition to supplying animals for investigations, also provided milk and meat including bacon. The road to the farm passed through a large village in which the three hundred or so junior staff of the Laboratory lived.

The Laboratory itself consisted of four divisions supported by a large administrative complex, which included a library, conference room and ample provision for the housing of records.

The Veterinary Training Division, which included a Veterinary School for training Veterinary Assistants, was also responsible for training Laboratory Technologists and so was largely Laboratory-based.

Staff in the Animal Production Division, which included a Parasitology Section, investigated the several problems caused by internal and external parasites of domestic animals, a reminder that many strange parasitic diseases of humans existed too. The nutritional requirements of the farm animals, mainly the dairy cattle, were also investigated. At the farm the poor milk yields of the indigenous Fulani cattle were upgraded by a cross-breeding programme. By artificial insemination using Friesian semen flown out from Britain, the cross-bred progeny gave more milk, but still enriched with the higher butter fat of the humped Zebu-type Fulani cattle.

Vaccines were produced by staff of the Bacteriology and Virology Divisions. There was no charge for the vaccines so they all had to be produced on a shoe-string budget.

Bacteriological vaccines, sent out in crown-corked beer bottles, protected cattle against Anthrax, Haemorrhagic Septicaemia and Blackquarter, called *'Harbin daji'* in Hausa (literally translated as 'The Arrow from the Bush'), because of the sudden onset of this fatal disease. The recipe for this vaccine began by making a meat digest using the natural enzyme, papain, found in green pawpaws, specially grown in a little grove near the laboratory. There were also two poultry vaccines, for Fowl Cholera and Fowl Typhoid, and also a vaccine against Bovine Pleuropneumonia.

Viral vaccines, freeze-dried to improve their storage qualities, were sent out in multi-dose ampoules. I was to become much more familiar with viral vaccines later, but 'new-chums' generally spent a short period in the Diagnostic Laboratory to familiarise themselves with some of the strange diseases which occurred locally.

Outside the Diagnostic Laboratory, near the aerogen plant which provided the gas used in the laboratory from air pumped through petrol, specimens from dead animals were collected at the adjacent autopsy area for later investigations in the laboratory. On the roof of the nearby building Hooded Vultures, *'Ungulu'* (or *Necrosyrtes monachus* if one preferred to roll their Latin name off the tongue), those ubiquitous scavengers which perform such a marvellous sanitary job in Africa, always lingered waiting for tit-bits.

Specimens were also received from Regional Laboratories or veterinary clinics all over Nigeria, generally sent in packed on ice by air, so that we received them fresh, and could culture them. Really out-of-way places on the far-flung borders of this large territory sent in preserved specimens.

No buses plied between Vom and Jos and the only passenger-carrying vehicles were lorries, or taxis mainly used by the wealthier Africans. These forms of public transport were hardly considered appropriate for expatriates, so I was encouraged to buy my own car under a government scheme which provided low-interest loans. A generous monthly allowance more than paid off the loan, if I was prepared to use my car on official government business. At the time I never realised how recently this privilege had been augmented. Only a year or two previously, expatriates in the lower ranks had to rely on bicycles or a weekly truck to Jos.

The lorries we saw frequently on the roads were colourfully decorated and identified in English or Hausa by names, mottos, religious exhortations or nicknames on a board over the cab. Some I recall – BLESS ME O GOD; CLANKING NELLIE; DESTINY IS INDELIBLE; OH! NIGERIA WHY WORRY; LORD NO BRAKES; FAITH HOPE AND CHARITY and GIVE US THIS DAY OUR DAILY BREAD. Had Roger been older, he could have made a fine collection of lorry names, in the manner of children making lists of railway engine types in Britain.

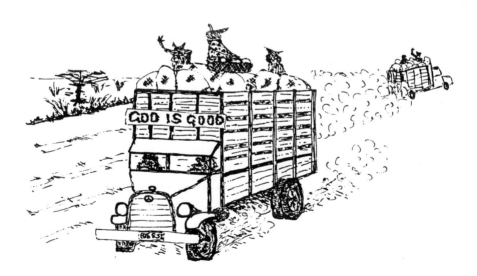

Mammy wagons

These lorries were usually piled high with all kinds of agricultural produce on which sat the passengers, mainly native women in their bright and colourful costumes; thus they were called 'Mammy wagons'. Dangerous and uncomfortable as a mode of transport, disaster usually struck when they got a wheel on the soft road shoulder during the wet season. They would cartwheel, scattering goods and passengers over several hundred feet. I was considerably sobered by one which went over a bridge parapet on the road to Jos. No passengers survived the twenty foot drop into the dry river bed, in spite of the lorry's battered nameplate declaring GOD IS GOOD.

My first trip into the bush, to a place called Dengi off the Plateau to the south-east, brought home to me how ignorant I was of local conditions and customs. Specimens submitted by the veterinary assistant in Dengi turned up something interesting and I felt it warranted a trip there to collect further material.

Not to be trusted on my own, I was assigned quite a retinue of staff to accompany me, no less than three veterinary assistants, two Mallam and an Alhaji, each wearing their flowing robe, or *Riga*. Quite determined to take Lassie and my gun for a bit of sport on the way, we all somehow squeezed into my roomy Morris Oxford, Lassie at the feet of the front passenger.

It was suggested I might like to spend the night at Dengi, but I was far too keen to get back to the fleshpots of Vom and quite sure we could do the round trip in a day, a mere 240 miles.

Gravel roads tended to get badly corrugated and rutted at the end of the wet season, so most drivers drove flat out; I was told the reason behind this was to save the shock absorbers or springs, but it did little to improve the mental anguish of passengers. Following the main road south to Pankshin, past the Panyam Fish Farm and through an impressive geological dyke near Mongu, I drove at a steady 60 m.p h. My passengers, strangely enough, seemed to have little to say.

Down the escarpment I slowed down a bit, for the road wound down through a drop of about 2,000 feet near Pankshin, but once at the bottom away we went again. In spite of mutterings from my passengers I was totally unprepared for the first river we encountered. I slowed a bit round a gentle double bend sloping downhill, wondering what the word DRIFT meant on a tattered roadside sign. Before I knew it or could slow further we were halfway across the forty metre wide river, stalled in a foot of water, steam billowing out from under the bonnet – 'Haba!'.

Lassie was the first to feel the water seeping into the car; she erupted from her place on the floor onto the seat beside me, showing little courtesy to my front seat passenger. We all got out hastily and waded to the far bank, the three dignified Hausa holding up their robes above their knees, giving me reproachful looks but saying little. No 'Rankai dade' I noticed. What should I do for an encore, I asked myself.

I was astonished how rapidly villagers appeared on the far bank. Hauling idiots out of the river was obviously their favourite pastime. In no time at all the car was manhandled out of the water, a bit wet on the floor inside and under the bonnet but otherwise perfectly all right, once the electrics were dried.

'Don't spoil the natives,' I had been told, so I very magnanimously gave one a shilling to share amongst themselves. Whatever they thought of me, they were far too polite to say anything. I later learnt that the going rate for being towed out ignominiously from a creek was a couple of pounds.

At Dengi not far away we attended to our business and set off home in good time, taking the drift very slowly. Perhaps I redeemed myself in the eyes of my companions, when a flock of Helmet Guinea Fowl had the temerity to cross the road in front of us just as we reached the bottom of the escarpment. Skidding to a stop and while my passengers looked on in astonishment, Lassie and I simultaneously erupted out of the car; she flushed them and I downed two – a left and right.

I was much more appreciative of local conditions and customs after my first rather abysmal performance in the bush. On subsequent trips I was allowed out alone (or perhaps no one was prepared to accompany me), but the journeys were not always trouble-free. A couple of years later I investigated an outbreak of rinderpest at the Lowlands Farm, a research station in the *Fadama* near Shendam, and nearly got caught in a grass fire.

Promoted to vaccine production a short while later, I was first allowed to practise my skills preparing Rabies vaccine for dogs and cats. This strain of Rabies virus, the Flury strain, had been adapted to grow in eggs by passaging it serially. Without going into the sordid details of the origin of the virus strain, the seed material was inoculated into the yolk sac of fertile eggs which had been incubated a week. They were candled daily, any dead ones discarded and ten days later the surviving embryos were collected, homogenised, filtered and the suspension squirted into ampoules in single-dog doses and freeze-dried. The batches were tested in mice and sometimes in guinea pigs. This vaccine was also my introduction to a long association with Rabies, performing and later supervising the diagnostic work on this common disease.

As Vom was situated within the tropics only a few degrees north of the equator, the hours of work were adjusted accordingly. In the Laboratory we normally started at 7.00 a.m., during the cool of the day; occasionally we started as early as 5.00 a.m. Because the houses were so close to our place of work we could go home for breakfast from 9.00 till 9.30. Work finished at 2.00, but on Saturdays we finished at noon and everyone then adjourned to the local club. Under the terms of our contract with the Colonial Office we were really supposed to be on call 24 hours a day, seven days a week. Colonial Regulations stated baldly that 'Officers are required to discharge the usual duties of the office to which they are appointed, and any other suitable duties which the Governor may call upon them to perform.' In fact there was always work outside these official hours. Frequently we enjoyed a leisurely stroll up to the Laboratory during the late afternoon to check on equipment or vaccines in preparation.

Around Vom open grassland stretched as far as the eye could see in most directions, denuded of trees by the demands of a charcoal industry which thrived in the past, particularly on the northern part of the Plateau. An equally demanding need for timber for hut poles and firewood had been recognised many years previously when eucalyptus trees, mainly the River Red Gum, *Eucalyptus camaldulensis*, were introduced first by Australian miners and later by the Forestry Department.

One of the most striking first impressions I had of Vom was the numerous tall gum trees of this species planted with great foresight many years previously. I was later to appreciate how the verdant nature of Vom, like an oasis in otherwise treeless grassland, attracted migrant birds passing through the area.

Rocky outcrops or *inselbergs* dotted the skyline, and a range of hills lay behind Vom Mission Hospital to the south of Vom. The larger alluvial tin-mining operations on the Plateau required plenty of water, so some large expanses of water lay nearby. Ouree Dam, west of Vom, provided water for a small hydro-electric power station near the foot of the escarpment on the west side of the Plateau. The Nigerian Electricity Supply Company (NESCO) supplied electricity to Vom, Jos and the many mining companies on the Plateau, their largest customers. They also had a much larger power station at Kurra Falls in the south-west of the Plateau.

When I first arrived, the surrounding countryside looked uninspiring bird-wise but matters improved considerably once the wet season got under way. Well-defined dry and wet seasons occurred on the Plateau. From October to March little rain fell and the *Harmattan*, a consistently cool but dry dusty wind from the Sahara, sometimes blew so strongly it cut the visibility so planes could not land at Jos airport. Temperatures rarely exceeded 90°F (32°C) and when the *Harmattan* was at its strongest the night temperature did at times fall below 32°F (0°C) because of the wind-chill factor and ice could be found on water containers exposed to the air. Swimming pools seemed icy-cold at that time of year. During the wet season some 60 inches (1500 mm) of rain fell over about six months with heavy thunderstorms and a few humid days at the beginning and end. In the wettest months, July and August, it became quite cool, justifying fires in the evenings; often the days were misty and dull.

During the late 1950s the only reference books on West African birds were lengthy tomes by Bannerman. It was not until 1960 that Elgood's small illustrated *Birds of the West African Town and Garden* became available. Bannerman's eight volume masterpiece and shorter two volume work represented all that was known on birds in West and Equatorial Africa. Most descriptions were drawn up from museum specimens, which required the bird in the hand for identification. Great gaps in knowledge existed on behaviour, preferred habitat, feeding and breeding. The illustrations were of little use for field identification.

By no stretch of the imagination could these weighty books be considered field guides. This was in an era before field guides became available. Thus I, and many like me, were considerably handicapped when it came to identifying the many strange new birds seen on walks around Vom. It largely became a matter of making notes then referring to the well-appointed library in the Laboratory, where some of Bannerman's works were available. At first I could not afford to buy a set of my own.

Unable to identify a bird from my rather sketchy notes, I sometimes got an identification of sorts from the several amateur naturalists with whom I was constantly meeting up, at the swimming pool, or over a beer in the club, or occasionally on my walks. Identification of the commoner birds around Vom was achieved by a gradual and endless absorption of knowledge through deduction and elimination.

Some species were unmistakable; large birds like the bustards and the Crowned Crane; colourful species like the weavers, bishops, whydahs, iridescent sunbirds, barbets, kingfishers and bee-eaters. Species, like the drab Kurrichane Thrush or the brighter Snowy-crowned Robin-chat, were secretive but had characteristic song. I listened to the monotonous 'Chip, Chip' of the Grey-backed Cameroptera for ages before I was able

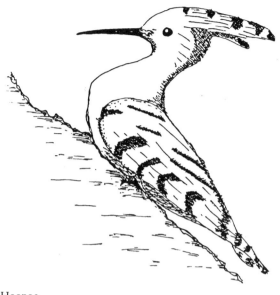

Hoopoe

to identify the bird. The Senegal Coucal, a large brown and white bird with black crown and red eye, made a strange noise, like water poured from a bottle, so was also known as the Bottle Bird. Barbary Shrikes, yellow-crowned and crimson-breasted, called in duet. The Plateau in the vicinity of Vom was indeed an ornithologist's paradise.

I was halfway through my first tour and just beginning to enjoy the work and social life in Vom and to get familiar with some of the birds of the Plateau when I was rather suddenly transferred to the Federal capital Lagos.

CHAPTER 2

Lagos and Bornu

IN LAGOS, THE FEDERAL CAPITAL OF NIGERIA, I found that I was the only veterinarian within some one hundred miles radius; even then Lagos had a population of over one million souls, and there were many expatriates with pets.

The Federal Department of Veterinary Research was one of two Federal organisations which had their headquarters outside Lagos. In our case all the members of our Directorate were in Vom except a rather hallowed administrator, 'The Permsec', who provided the link between Director and Minister and whom I rarely had the pleasure of meeting. Amongst the lower echelons a professional officer had to be present in the Federal capital to attend to the more mundane veterinary matters. At short notice I had been selected to relieve the incumbent veterinary research officer, Duthie Slater, who was spending six months on study leave.

The job seemed to be simple enough: Run an office and supervise a small veterinary clinic at Obalende on Lagos island: Attend to all export matters: Show the flag at several government farms nearby. However I was not at all happy about this temporary move, though I knew better than to argue the toss too much.

My first nine months in Vom had undoubtedly spoilt me. On the Plateau the climate, the availability of fresh vegetables and food, the pleasant company and working conditions were very different from what I found in Lagos. The high coastal humidity sapped my energy; the working hours were officially from 8.00 a.m. to 2.00 p.m. straight through, by which time I had lost any appetite for lunch; as a result I also lost a lot of weight. Thus I found it hard to comprehend the attitude of expatriates living in Lagos, who liked the big city with all its amenities and reacted with disgust, even horror, at the possibility of being transferred up north or to the Plateau.

Before I even moved to Lagos, the instructions I received in Vom conflicted with my professional conscience. It was carefully explained to me that I was not to get too involved with the work of the Obalende veterinary clinic, which was run by a capable veterinary assistant, James Adeleye. House-calls were not to be made. Unfortunately this had not been explained to the many expatriates who insisted on seeing me about their pets. Several were very unreasonable and demanding. They assumed that I was in Lagos for their benefit only and some even had the gall to pester me at home.

How unreasonable some people could be was brought home to me soon after I moved to Lagos and took over, when I had a phone call from miles away late one evening at my bungalow. I was abruptly commanded to collect a Labrador which had died of the terminal nervous stages of distemper. I knew James Adeleye had been treating the unfortunate animal without much success for some days. As compassionately as possible I explained to the owner, who it seemed occupied some high position in the Department of Prisons, that I had been instructed not to make house calls, but would try and arrange collection early the next morning. He became abusive, making me wonder where my first brush with the law would land me, and later wrote several angry letters including, I believe, one to the Royal College of Veterinary Surgeons in London, complaining about my lack of interest. I hope that illustrious body treated his letter with the contempt it deserved. I explained my side of the story in a letter to my Director, Ian Taylor, and heard nothing more about this unfortunate episode. My letter also allowed me to get in a sly dig at the hierarchy, for I had not been reimbursed expenses incurred in my move from Vom and was broke.

Veterinary surgeons know full well it is not the pets but their owners who often cause the most trouble. Where I had time, I generally tried to attend to their pets when approached personally, providing it did not interfere with my other duties. Of course, being a government officer, I was not allowed to charge for such services, though I believe a previous government veterinary officer in Lagos had built up a thriving and lucrative but illicit practice.

Having enjoyed the clinical aspects of veterinary work in Britain and on rare occasions in Vom, I found it frustrating in Lagos to spend a great deal of my time signing export certificates or showing my face at the several government establishments in the vicinity like the nearby poultry farm and dairy, the cattle lairage and, early in the morning once a month, the slaughter-house. The meat inspectors there were quite capable of detecting the signs of major zoonotic diseases in the cattle carcases, like parasitic cysts or infections, but my 'showing-the-flag' visits to the abattoir required a departure from my house soon after midnight in order to negotiate the traffic which seemed even worse at night.

A veterinary philosopher once said 'The quack is judged by his successes, the professional man by his failures.' Strangely I had some successes, but what astonished me most was how sometimes the simplest approach or treatment could produce the most dramatic result. There was the case of the parrot with the broken leg, for instance.

A rather amiable high court judge phoned me in my office one day in great distress to say that his West African Grey Parrot, a pet of many years, had caught its foot in the cage and broken its leg. If it wasn't too much trouble, would I put it to sleep. This variety of parrot was highly prized and this individual spoke well, but had little to say while I examined the tarsus which in the parrot family is a short bone. X-ray facilities we did not have, but it seemed a clean break and the foot was hanging sideways. Fortunately the skin was unbroken and I was able to straighten the bone and tape a strip of plaster round the straightened leg, with pieces of matchstick as a splint. When I removed the plaster later the bird had made a perfect recovery and I earned the undying gratitude of its owner.

Another case involved a dachshund. The little sausage-dog's owner, whom I got to know on my late afternoon walks with Lassie, worked in aviation and lived in a palatial two storey mansion not far from our modest bungalow. One afternoon I was invited in for a beer – there was a catch of course. Soon after making myself comfortable I was told,

'Poor little Snags collapsed yesterday – she's in a coma and Adeleye can't do anything. Would you have a look at her please?' It was the 'please' which did it.

Vital signs were barely there, for she looked just about dead, with very shallow respirations and a very weak pulse. She did not look like a case of rabies, my first consideration. I felt there was nothing to lose by giving her an intravenous stimulant and without finishing my beer I returned to my bungalow to collect my bag. Like Lazarus, she rose after my injection and was still behaving normally several weeks later. Perhaps it was some obscure nervous condition, or unknown insect-borne viral encephalitis, or heatstroke. I still do not know what had been the matter with her.

Quantities of hides and skins were exported to Europe from Apapa docks, the port of Lagos, and all consignments had to be certified free of disease. I was reluctant to sign certificates sight unseen and thereby expose myself to the risk of being struck off the veterinary register. Besides, just looking at the hides would not have told me much. The solution lay in the way they had been treated. They were sun-dried and then treated with arsenic, and it was generally agreed that this treatment would kill most of the infectious agents, of which anthrax and foot-and-mouth virus were the most serious. Thus I signed cautiously-worded certificates which included the clause . . . *believed to be free of disease, by virtue of their treatment,* but only after the exporters had certified that the hides had been properly treated.

Dare I admit that following the subsequent discovery of Anthrax spores in the skin-dyeing vats at Kano, some hides and skins tested later in Vom did reveal some rather alarming results, which were not widely publicised. The relatively high incidence of Anthrax around the port of Liverpool, where Nigerian hides were unloaded along with hides from other countries like India and Pakistan, has often been noted in the veterinary press.

Visits to the lairage two or three times weekly, a sandy waste beyond the railway terminus on the mainland, necessitated negotiating the dreadful bottleneck of traffic jams on Carter Bridge. Cattle were held at the lairage very temporarily pending export to neighbouring territories in trucks. At first no ramps were available for loading or unloading cattle. Trucks were loaded in the crudest possible manner. The long-horned Zebu cattle were positioned against the lowered tailboard of the truck and many willing hands lifted the tailboard, beast and all, into the back in a jumbled tangle of legs and horns, accompanied by exclamations and exhortations – '*Hamdala . . .! Yauwa . . .!*' I felt the least I could do to facilitate the loading of these unfortunate beasts was to expedite the installation of a proper loading ramp which my predecessor had already designed.

Thinking there was nothing demanding about these simple duties expected of me, I was brought down to earth with a thump when I diagnosed Foot and Mouth Disease (FMD) in a piggery alongside the only route into the cattle lairage. My immediate thought on that Friday morning was 'Why are these things sent to try us at the end of the week?' The infected pigs were of little concern once they were slaughtered, but the problem was what to do about the cattle. Like the hides and skins, cattle awaiting export to the neighbouring countries of Senegal and Ghana had to be certified free of a number of diseases including FMD; neither country wanted cattle that might be carrying disease, so all exports temporarily ceased. There was no grazing for the cattle and little fodder available. They could not be moved elsewhere except for slaughter. As usual *Bature* was expected to come up with some miraculous solution to this seemingly unsolvable problem. All I could do was stop further cattle arriving from the north and go off to friends in Ibadan, a convenient hundred miles or so up the road, for a prearranged weekend with the family.

These family weekends were very rare occasions indeed, for the only-veterinary-surgeon-within-a-hundred-miles was automatically made Honorary Veterinary Surgeon to the Lagos Race Club. For a small honorarium I, accompanied by James Adeleye, attended every race meeting, even during the long weekend holidays. The Lagos Polo Club tried hard to cajole me also, but only succeeded once, when I attended a match against Accra in May. On the programme list of officials I appeared amongst a Major-General and two Colonels, and was grateful they had omitted my army rank. My father, who had played polo in India, would have appreciated the game more.

The race meetings were noisy and exciting, but no broken bones, thank goodness, or even bad falls for that matter. However, the Stewards were eager to curb any doping which might be going on and briefed me accordingly.

The Easter race meeting in 1958 as usual went on for several days and I found myself unwittingly drawn into a pioneer event in the history of the Club. As a highlight to this meeting the Stewards announced beforehand that they had decided to institute anti-doping measures; all winners were to be swabbed. Under the watchful eyes of several thousand spectators, James and I did our bit, taking saliva swabs in the winner's enclosure with all the precautions I knew were necessary.

It really made my day when all returned positive swabs. Herd & Munday, the analytical chemists in Britain, to whom all the carefully collected swabs were sent by air freight, detected caffeine in every swab.

The stewards were still trying to unravel this mystery when I finished my time in Lagos, but my explanation was that caffeine was one of the active constituents of the kola nut and I believe thin slivers were fed to the horses for good luck. The ubiquitous kola nut was used by the Africans, like the betel leaf in India, as a stimulant, but was also offered to friends as a gesture of friendship.

My title of Veterinary Research Officer seemed redundant in Lagos. I could find precious little research to do in my rather mundane job. One place I visited several times to satisfy my cravings for a bit of erudite knowledge was Yaba on the mainland where medical laboratories and the West African Council for Medical Research (WACMR) were located.

On my first visit to WACMR, where some of the pioneer work on Yellow Fever was performed, I was ushered into a small cubicle where a microscope was set up. My guide reverently pointed to the specimen and announced, 'Noguchi's liver' – he pronounced it as written and I hoped he took my expression of stunned misunderstanding for one of great interest, for I did not want to show my ignorance by asking, 'Who on earth was Noguchi?' Twenty-five years later on a visit to Hideyo Noguchi's museum on the shores of Lake Inawashiro near Koriyama in Japan, I then realised he was an eminent Japanese microbiologist of an earlier era who died of Yellow Fever in West Africa; some believed he experimentally infected himself. At WACMR work on Yellow Fever was still proceeding and some baboons had been infected. I was invited to watch a liver biopsy taken from an adult baboon. Seemingly no pre-medication or sedation was offered to the poor beast, which was pinioned by a brawny assistant while the operator took his sample, his face only inches from the gnashing fangs. Rather him than me, I agreed.

At our first meeting, the entomologist at WACMR, John Boorman, took me home in his car, during which trip his dog vomited all over my shoes. Though I met John many times subsequently even up in Vom and greatly admired his prolific articles on insects in the Journal of the Nigerian Field Society, one on the Hawkmoths of Nigeria was superb, it is strange how one is remembered. Fifteen years later when John was working at the Virus Research Institute, Pirbright in England, I visited that famous institution and bumped into him at the entrance to the showers. Obviously trying hard to put a name to me, he blurted out, 'I remember you, my dog was sick all over you!'

The small bungalow we occupied in the pleasant suburb of Ikoyi was on an island, not far from the creek along the banks of which we would stroll most evenings and let Lassie lie in the water amongst a myriad hermit crabs. The low lying nature of Ikoyi Island was brought home to us when the wet season started and our garden became inundated.

Our neighbours used a boat to get to the road and the deafening frog chorus every night kept us awake.

Around the bungalow several palm trees were of the kind that were tapped for palm wine. The tapper would periodically appear and his activities always seemed to intrigue Roger, who knew the fairytale of *Jack and the Beanstalk* – perhaps he wondered why the giant never chased the tapper down the tree. The tapper collected the sap from the crown, the terminal inflorescence, into beer bottles. After climbing up and down the tall palms using a rope loop, he poured the liquid into large gourds hung on either side of the back wheel of his bicycle

Unfermented, the fresh sap tasted watery and sweetish, but after a day or two it commenced bubbling and became more potent the longer it was left to brew. *Pagal pani* or 'Fool water' it was called in India, and I have no doubt the local vintage was as strong, though I could never pluck up the courage to sample the seemingly revolting bubbling brew.

Kuramo Waters, a lagoon ideal for young children, and Victoria Beach were readily approachable by canoe or vehicle for bathing. Years later the same beach offered more spectacular entertainment when executions by firing squad were carried out there.

The huge sprawling metropolis of Lagos stretched over several islands and the adjacent mainland to which it was joined by a causeway and by the older Carter Bridge, often jammed with traffic even in those days. Dominant over the skyline near the bridge was the Powerhouse near the railway station at Iddo. The main shopping centre and Kingsway supermarket catered for the expatriates but a huge sprawling market extended along the roadside. The airport at Ikeja was some fifteen miles north.

Of reptiles we saw plenty, though not many snakes. Geckos hid behind furnishings in the house and came out at night to carefully stalk moths and insects around the lights. Lassie chased bright orange and blue male *Agama* or Rainbow lizards everywhere.

However of birds I saw very few species. I can recall a pair of shikras nesting in a tall tree behind the house. I derived a lot of pleasure from watching these dashing small hawks. They brought a regular supply of small unidentifiable birds and lizards to their young. Otherwise there seemed to be little to observe apart from the ubiquitous vultures, pigeons, crows and weaver birds. Perhaps this was one of the rare occasions in my life when I let my work interfere with my pleasures.

After my spell in Lagos, the family flew back directly to Britain, but I returned to Vom by rail, taking Lassie with me but leaving my car with the Public Works Department, the Fiddle-de-dee, in Lagos.

I was not due leave for another two months. It was hardly worthwhile getting back into vaccine production for such a short time, so I was asked to go up to Bornu Province in the north-east of Nigeria, ostensibly to demonstrate a new test for Bovine Pleuropneumonia to the staff in the regional laboratory in Maiduguri, but also to have a good look at the field veterinary services and do a bit of touring – 'go to bush,' was the term for it.

Provided with a Landrover and driver, I took along Dantiyi, my shotgun and a fine assortment of borrowed touring kit. Lassie remained with friends in Vom. The departmental vehicles were always provided with a driver-mechanic and we were discouraged from driving them. During the middle of the wet season many roads were impassable and closed, so I was issued with a barrier-pass. Once in Bornu I soon saw the reason. On one stretch of road we took about six hours to cover forty miles of black cotton soil, churning along in low-ratio, four-wheel drive. The flooding was dramatic, as the flat countryside drained imperceptibly towards the north-east into the Lake Chad basin.

There were huge flocks of wildfowl and I did some useful shooting for the pot. Several spur-winged geese I downed, but they were as tough as old boots with much the same flavour. However knob-billed and pygmy geese and duck, especially the ubiquitous *Wishi-wishi* were more palatable. When we sickened of wildfowl there were always fish, huge Niger perch -*Giwan ruwa* – literally 'water-elephant' – to be bought locally.

I enjoyed the six weeks or so in the field, mainly in the company of the Provincial Veterinary Officer, Dickie Knowles, learning a lot and imbibing a lot too, during the long evenings. He seemed to think I had too much blood in my alcohol.

We visited several veterinary clinics in villages where there was inevitably a tall tree full of nesting egrets and weavers. We walked round newly-built slaughter slabs where vultures outnumbered the slaughtermen; we looked at hide-drying facilities; we stayed in some comfortable bush rest-houses, spaced out in the pre-war era a comfortable day's walk or ride apart. Many bush rest-houses in the north had an avocado tree or two nearby; one veterinary officer, Dennis Walker, planted them

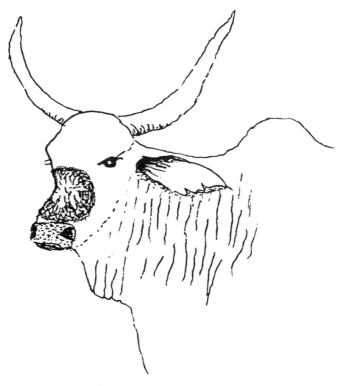

Fulani Cow – 'Dashe'

everywhere he went. Around the rest-houses *Neem* trees from India provided dense shade.

With the approaching dry season some cattle herds were ready to move into the river basins, the areas infested with tsetse fly, the carrier of Trypanosomiasis. In cattle, this was a wasting disease unlike the human form of sleeping sickness. A new prophylactic drug protected the cattle for several months while in an infected area. The Fulani paid for THE RED MEDICINE as they called it. At one camp I visited, veterinary assistants were injecting each animal into the muscles of its hindquarters as it was roped and brought forward while a Danish veterinary officer, Ole Karst, stood on an anthill in the middle of a milling mass of cattle, and estimated the dose for each animal by guessing their body weight.

One mob of cattle I saw were infected with Bovine Pleuropneumonia. The animals were segregated from the main cattle routes and held in quarantine. Their owner was offered vaccine but instead chose the crude old-fashioned way of immunising them – *Dashe* – by scarifying their noses with virulent exudate from a dead infected animal. What the

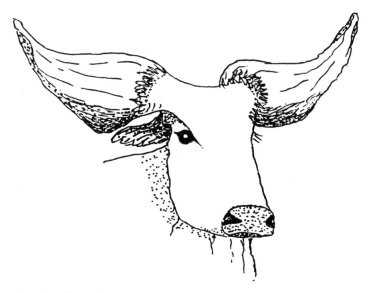

Kuri Cow from Lake Chad.

34

treatment did not kill it cured, but the resultant huge erosive ulcers left little of the face.

At the markets were Kuri cattle from Lake Chad with huge bulbous hollow horns, whose weight was supposed to tip back their heads and keep their noses out of water as they swam between islands. The huge surface area of the horns may also play a part in temperature regulation, assisting in heat loss. On the road hornbills with huge hollow bills frequently flew across the roads in front of the vehicle looking like 'Droop-snoots' – their bills so like the sloped-down noses of one of the latest airforce fighters and later the Concorde.

All too soon it was time to return to Vom and then proceed on leave. On the eve of our departure from Damaturu, I went down to the *Fadama*, the grassy floodplain of the river, for a last look at the wildfowl. A spur-winged goose came too close, tempting providence, and I shot it, donating the large bird to the driver.

The following morning as we motored up the Panshanu Pass onto the Plateau heading back to Vom, having spent the night in Bauchi, I stopped the driver for a last lingering look into the blue distance back the way we had come. I became aware of the most appalling smell seemingly emanating from beneath the bonnet of the overheated Landrover, as if all the rubber hoses had caught fire. The driver insisted *'Ba kome shi ke nan'* – 'Everything's fine.' Nevertheless I decided to have a look and he sheepishly lifted the bonnet. Draped over the hot engine block and exhaust manifold were strips of blackened goose flesh, a novel method of barbequeing his meal on our way home.

I ended my first tour by returning to Britain on a Dutch cargo boat, the M. S. *Gabonkust*, one of the Holland-West-Africa Line's vessels. This tranquil way of travelling appealed to me, so before leaving Lagos to tour the north-east I made all the necessary arrangements. I flew from Vom to Lagos to join her.

The relaxed atmosphere and good food on board restored my weight, though I had an anxious moment when confronted with my first meal of raw minced steak, a Dutch delicacy, which I found quite delicious too, but only after I was assured the steak had not been purchased in Nigeria.

For most of the voyage I was the only passenger, with a stateroom to myself. I read a lot and saw one French movie several times; otherwise the only shipboard entertainment was provided at ports along the coast where cargo was taken on from surfboats. I was reminded that this precarious method of loading and unloading in a heavy swell had been the lot of 'Old Coasters' in the pre-war years even at Lagos, before Apapa docks were completed. The few ladies in those days were lifted in a sort of bosun chair called a 'Mammy chair.'

Sea passages were in great demand either way because, with Government officers, leave did not commence until reaching Liverpool. A new tour did not commence until back in Nigeria. We were encouraged to fly by being offered an extra week's leave either way.

I was fortunate to get a sea trip back to Nigeria for the family in March 1959 on the M. V. *Accra*, a very comfortable ship which provided many different forms of shipboard entertainment, so different from what I had experienced on the M. S. *Gabonkust* only four months before. The sea passage allowed me to exploit a loophole I found in the Customs Department legislation. An old Act allowing officers in pre-war days to take out sufficient non-perishable food in 'Chop boxes' to last a complete tour had never been rescinded. 'Chop' was food, which was always 'passed' not served. 'Small chop' usually referred to canapes or 'finger food.'

Through useful family connections, we were able to buy cartons at wholesale prices in England, so arrived in Lagos with several large cartons of 'chop' and a handful of papers with which I was able to confuse the customs officer who dealt with us. After much deliberation he passed the lot. We thus saved quite a lot of money as prices in Nigeria were generally higher.

June and Roger, accompanied by some eighteen bits of assorted luggage and large cartons, travelled from Lagos to Vom by rail. I had to collect my car, but when I arrived at the 'Fiddle-de-Dee' yard in Lagos before it was ready, I was astonished to find the bright red leather upholstery had grown a delicate green mould, like velvet, which took time to remove. But for this delay I might have beaten the train to Vom. As it was I covered the 680 miles from Lagos to Vom, mostly on red laterite unsealed roads, in a day and a half.

The last 500 miles took a hot, sweaty, dusty fourteen hours over some parts of the main road which were badly corrugated. Leaving Ilorin at daybreak, I crossed the River Niger at Jebba Bridge, the single track also shared by the railway. I dined on fresh fruit from wayside stalls, but had no time to dally at Bida to admire their manufactured glass ornaments or at Abuja to look at their traditional pottery. In one native village, through the narrow back streets of which I drove slowly, I was undeterred by a very agile goat, which leapt out of a doorway onto the bonnet of

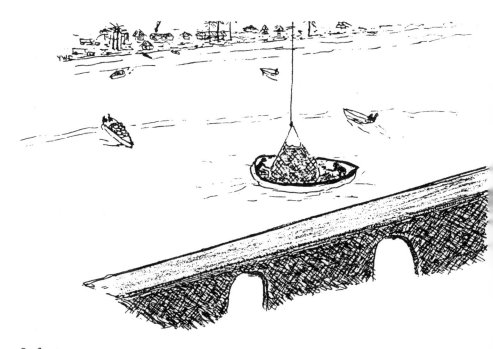

Surfboats

37

my Morris, and from there into the open doorway of a house opposite, apparently unharmed.

Crossing the Kaduna River, a tributary of the River Niger, on a ferry, I reached Assob Falls at the foot of the Plateau escarpment just after dusk. From there the road was sealed and the cooler air on the climb up to the Plateau in the dark was a wonderful relief.

CHAPTER 3

Vom 1959 –
Animal Vaccines and Birds

IT SEEMED CUSTOMARY AFTER A DINNER PARTY FOR THE HOST TO INVITE GUESTS 'TO SEE AFRICA' – a strange custom whereby the men folk wandered outside to water the flowers and make appropriate comments about the wide and starry night, while the ladies powdered their noses using the facilities inside. I recall on one such occasion an encounter with driver ants, which enlivened the proceedings. These marauding ants, also known as soldier or army ants, were particularly active at the change of seasons when the humid days made them more invasive; they cleaned up everything before them. If they invaded the kitchen or house one could be sure they would clean out all the cockroaches and it was best to leave them to it, provided all pets were moved out of their way. Their drones were the ubiquitous sausage flies, which clumsily flew around lights at night. The Africans ate them.

Ants were but one of the many species of creepy-crawlies with which we had to contend. Large bird-eating spiders, millipedes, scarab (dung) beetles of all shapes and sizes, scorpions and bees – the emphasis was on them being African KILLER bees – were inevitably encountered by new families as part of their African initiation.

During my second tour we were delighted to be able to participate more in the social life on the Plateau. Dinner parties and musical evenings became regular occurrences. At these functions it was quite in order for young children, already in their night clothes, to be taken along and laid on the host's bed under the mosquito net. At the end of the evening they were collected, slumbering peacefully, and carried to the car to be taken home. Roger was not at all amused when I once stumbled and deposited him in a flowerbed.

June and I even started to play bridge once or twice a week, but not very seriously as we enjoyed more the chatty evenings with the Chifneys. There were also Clubs which we could join. Vom club was mainly a watering hole when we first arrived, with a bar and billiard table. Later the building was expanded to accommodate the productions of our flourishing amateur dramatic society, Vom Players, which attracted audiences from afar. At a squeeze the enlarged club could accommodate audiences of about 120 and we often played to packed houses. June and I enjoyed taking small parts in these productions.

On the Plateau two larger clubs, with swimming pools and a variety of facilities including weekly film shows, were run by the Amalgamated Tin Mines of Nigeria, ATMN for short, the largest tin-mining company in Nigeria. Although mainly for their staff, both the Yelwa Club nearby in Bukuru and the other about fifteen miles south at Barakin Ladi were open to all expatriates. A swim at Yelwa Club followed by a curry lunch became very much part of our lives on Sundays.

Now entrenched in the Virology Division, with little likelihood of being sent away again, having satisfactorily completed my penance in Lagos, I was able to learn more about the viral vaccines produced in the Division. They were all live attenuated vaccines, that is, modified to provoke a mild form of the disease and a lasting immunity.

By far the most important viral disease of cattle was rinderpest, known also as Cattle Plague, a highly fatal disease spread by fairly close contact between infected animals. The viruses causing rinderpest of cattle, distemper of dogs and measles of humans are closely related serologically, in fact strange innovative tests were once in vogue, using tests, say, for distemper to detect rinderpest antibodies in cattle. There was even a hint of cross protection; rinderpest-infected meat protected hounds against distemper; an interesting observation, indeed, yet hardly practical.

In the 1920s the only known means of protecting cattle against rinderpest was the simultaneous administration of virulent virus and immune serum, which sometimes produced unpredictable results. Later an inactivated (killed) vaccine was tried but only conferred immunity for a short period. By the late 1950s two live attenuated vaccines were available.

Lapinised Rinderpest Vaccine (LRV) was prepared in rabbits but did not travel well. It was a messy vaccine to produce and was only used in breeds of cattle which were highly susceptible to rinderpest, such as the dwarf humpless cattle in the south, the N'dama and Muturu breeds. Strangely, these breeds, which lived in the forested Tsetse-fly belt, were highly resistent to Trypanosomiasis.

The other vaccine was Caprinised Rinderpest Vaccine, generally referred to as Dried Goat Virus (DGV), which at first conjured up in my mind visions of the whole goat being minced up, though in fact only its spleen was used. Even in the humped Zebu cattle, those owned by the nomadic Fulani, this vaccine caused a fever and sometimes aggravated bowel infections, but conferred a lasting immunity. Strangely the febrile reaction could be used beneficially if there was doubt that a consignment of vaccine had been mishandled in transit, for instance left in the sun on the concrete apron at an airport, a not infrequent occurrence. A few cattle at the destination would be inoculated with the suspect batch of vaccine and if they reacted with a temperature the batch was considered still satisfactory.

Having spent part of my childhood at Naini Tal in the Himalayan foothills not far from the Imperial Institute of Veterinary Research at Mukteswar in India, I was fascinated by this vaccine which was developed there by Edwards in the 1920s about the time I was born. He serially passaged virulent rinderpest virus in goats many times and showed that it became fixed; in the process the virus became modified or attenuated for cattle. Considered a serendipitous accident at the time, scientists later were to attribute the change of character of the virus to the selection of a temperature-sensitive mutant during the multiple passaging in goats.

This most famous vaccine in the era of steam-age virology, must have been used to immunise countless millions of cattle in tropical areas of the world where rinderpest existed. It was a relatively simple vaccine to produce as unskilled junior staff could be used to their utmost capacity, but was becoming increasingly unacceptable because of the high proportion of adverse reactions.

Because of this, research on the development of a milder rinderpest vaccine, like Nakamura's avianised-lapinised vaccine, was in progress when I first arrived in Vom, but seemed to be a very fiddly vaccine to produce. Taking out goat spleens was one thing; trying to find the spleens of chick embryos seemed to be a much harder undertaking.

Three years later I was to be involved with the production and field assessment of a tissue-cultured rinderpest vaccine. Long before then, however, in fact soon after I started my second tour, there was an urgent demand for a vaccine suitable for Zebu cattle believed to be highly susceptible because of their isolation. Along the eastern border of Nigeria with neighbouring Cameroon, were a series of isolated plateaus, of which the most well-known was the Mambila Plateau, where several thousand Fulani cattle found excellent grazing. It was necessary to protect these cattle along the border where a rinderpest outbreak smouldered. DGV was considered much too severe. LRV it would have to be, but this vaccine being so fragile it was doubted whether it could be sent to this Plateau without spoiling on the way, because there was no airport conveniently nearby, in fact not even a motorable road providing access, and all vaccines and other supplies would have to be carried up by porter. An inactivated (killed) vaccine was a third possibility considered.

Near Jos, the original rinderpest immunisation camp set up in the 1920s was at a place called Mai-idon-toro. I believe the site was originally owned by a tin miner with very small eyes or perhaps a glass eye. *Idon-toro* translates as 'eye like a threepenny coin.' The Northern Region Veterinary Department later acquired this place to house their Regional Veterinary Officer. A group of us from Vom – I only went along for the ride – inspected the old buildings with a view to producing an inactivated vaccine, using virulent rinderpest virus which could not be safely handled at Vom where it might contaminate the other rinderpest vaccines. To go back to such an early technique seemed a retrogressive step to my elementary way of thinking, but who was I to offer an opinion, not that I was asked anyway.

I am pleased to say that ingenuity prevailed. The veterinary officer covering the Mambila Plateau, Iain MacFarlane, had kerosene refrigerators set up every few miles along the steep pathway to produce plenty of ice. Porters carried insulated boxes containing ampoules of LRV packed in ice up the tortuous track. The cattle were vaccinated, I presume successfully, since no serious outbreak occurred.

I was already familiar with Rabies Vaccine production for dogs and cats, but vaccines were also produced to protect village poultry against Fowl Pox (FP) and Newcastle Disease (ND), a very prevalent and fatal disease. In India ND is called Ranikhet Disease, after the small hill town of Ranikhet, near Naini Tal and Mukteswar, where their first outbreak occurred.

ND vaccine was prepared in Vom from the Komarov strain of virus. Administered by injection into the muscle of the leg, it caused paralysis in some birds and was not acceptable for use in the intensive poultry industry which was only just starting. For them research was being conducted on milder vaccines which could be simply administered to chicks as a drop in their eye or in drinking water, thus minimising handling of the birds.

The old house, into which we moved soon after starting my second tour, was situated on the north side of Vom surrounded by more than an acre of garden. Apart from absences on leave we retained this house for the remainder of our time in Vom. Built during the war, the bungalow was austere but surprisingly comfortable, with concrete floors and a wooden ceiling. The galvanised tin roof was noisy when it rained. The plumbing was rather archaic. Windows were thief-proofed with XPM, an expanded metal grill. The heavy P.W.D. furniture was built to last. Off the main bedroom a door led to the back verandah and we learnt

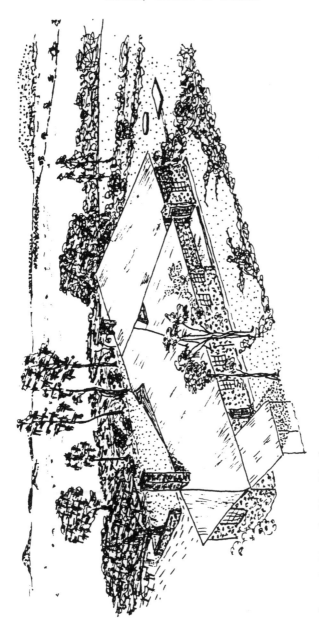

Our house in Vom, looking North

it was called the Fulani door. Ours was one of the last houses to be built with such a convenience. When wives were not encouraged in the country, some husbands took a native mistress; Fulani women were considered attractive. The quarters for our household staff were at a discreet distance out the back.

Around the front of our stone-built house, a dense bed of dahlias six feet high, attracted sunbirds, nectar-feeding birds of the family *Nectariniidae*, which I was encountering for the first time. Like the humming-birds of the New World and the honey-eaters of Australia, they fill a niche that does not seem to exist in Britain or Europe.

The front garden was a wilderness of shrubs set amongst eucalyptus trees of medium height, which provided shade. Around the house an open drain diverted water from the bath and basins and the roof run-off into a soakwell. Water lying in little puddles in this drain attracted many smaller birds, mannikins, fire-finches and cordon-bleus. Considered rather primitive by modern-day standards, this open drain had its uses and later I built a hydroponicum to utilise this relatively clean source of water and grew very fine tomatoes. Near the house it was an unwritten rule that one prevented pools of stagnant water from collecting, as they provided breeding grounds for mosquito larvae. For this reason there was a regulation that bananas could not be grown near houses because of water which might collect in the deep leaf insertions.

However our side garden contained several mature citrus fruit trees and a large mango tree, into which I watched a small finch, a red-cheeked cordon bleu, carrying wisps of grass, obviously building a nest. All too eager to try out my nest-finding capabilities in our new garden, I later climbed up to check the completed nest in the tree top, not aware that this little bird frequently built close to a paper wasp's nest for mutual protection. I was stung three times on my ear and almost fell out of the tree, providing great entertainment for a group of village children who were surveying the tree with more serious intent. In spite of this tree producing stringy fruit strongly flavoured with turpentine, the young village kids loved them. Frequently Lassie treed a few children, thinking it all a huge joke, barking madly, with her tail going like a metronome.

Once Lassie was called to heel the children would descend sheepishly and scuttle off – *'Sannu Bature'* – but be back again next day.

Too much work makes Jack a dull boy. There were plenty of extra-mural activities to get involved with outside the Laboratory. Golf, with which I had a transient love affair, tennis, squash, horse-riding, swimming, sailing were all readily available on the Plateau.

We, and of course Lassie, preferred to walk out into the surrounding countryside where we found plenty of places to explore. I soon became one of those eccentric expatriates, of whom there seemed to be many, who cultivated an interest in the native flora, fauna or customs. Most well-known amongst the Vom residents, Veterinary School Principal, Robert Gambles – *'Ungulu'* – became a world authority on West African Dragonflies and was often seen walking with an enormous butterfly net over his shoulders.

A favoured haunt of ours, an *Inselberg* called Kafo Rock, was situated only a mile away along a rough but motorable track. Amongst the rocks at Kafo a depression flooded during the wet season and was known as The Wishi Pool, because White-faced Whistling Teal were often seen there; they were called *Wishi-wishi* in Hausa, after their call. They were common, tame and as a result easily shot, incapable of the aerial ma-noeuvres which make the European Teal such a hard target. They were generally shot all through the year but early in the 1959 wet season I shot an adult at this pool. I was considerably upset to find young ducklings on the water nearby, which prompted me to impose my own close season on these ducks during the wet season. I was by no means the first or last to do so, for these birds were so easily approached when they were nesting.

I shot mainly for the pot because meat of any sort was a welcome addition to our diet. Although we could buy pork, ham or chicken from our farm, and sometimes very tasty beef when a feeding trial was completed at the LIC, our main source of protein was mutton or goat.

Joints were brought round to the door still twitching in a bucket, a rather revolting sight, although the carcases were inspected routinely by a veterinarian to ensure they were free of any horrible disease or parasitic infection.

Other gamebirds also found around Vom, like Double-spurred Francolin (Bushfowl) and bustard, the commonest being the Black-bellied Bustard, were generally elusive and could only be flushed with a dog. Lassie was usually out of control when trailing their scent and put them up far ahead, so everything was in favour of the birds. They also nested during the wet season.

Great Snipe migrated through Nigeria during August each year, and during a brief fortnight or so they could be found in the wetter paddocks around Vom. They provided good sport during the wet season and were considered fair game, generally sitting tight. When flushed, often with difficulty, their flight was not as erratic as the Common Snipe. They also had more flesh on them, and during my early years in Vom I shot several. They provided a toothsome morsel when wrapped in bacon and grilled, after plucking and cleaning out their insides.

I was never game to try cooking them as my father had described when he had shot Pintail Snipe on the snipe *Jheels* in India. His recipes were simple: EITHER wrap in mud, feathers and all, bake in an open fire for a few minutes, then peel them; OR pluck, hold by the beak and dip into boiling butter in a deep container for twenty seconds. By either method one was expected to eat them, bones, guts and all.

A marked seasonal appearance of many species of birds provided evidence of considerable local movement. For instance Carmine bee-eaters suddenly appeared at the start of the dry season and were seen particularly at grass fires where they fed on insects; they bred elsewhere on the major rivers. Vinaceous Turtle-doves also appeared then, their staccato and persistent call 'Better-go-home' was heard all around. The Grey-headed or Chestnut-bellied Kingfisher appeared at the end of the dry season, starting to breed immediately by excavating their nestholes in the eroded banks of a water-course – *Kurmi* – or roadside pit.

Well before the end of the wet season the grasslands suddenly became

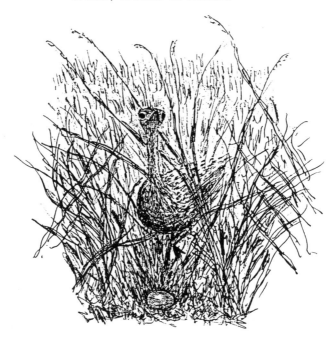

Black-bellied Bustard's nest, not easy to find or photograph

alive with many male Orange Bishops flitting about in their territories, strikingly handsome in their black and red breeding plumage. Present throughout the year, this species did not migrate, but the males in their non-breeding plumage looked just like females, so they were overlooked. Other species of weavers behaved in the same way, but were less common. Male Napoleon Bishops and Yellow-mantled Whydahs, or Widow-birds, were resplendent in black and gold. During my second tour of duty in Vom I started putting names to many of the local species of birds and made interesting discoveries about their habits.

I soon learnt that in the tropics different groups of birds bred at different times of the year: Vom lay only 9 degrees north of the Equator. As there was not much variation in the length of the day throughout the year, breeding was not triggered by the lengthening days which occur in the spring in more temperate climates, but more by the availability of food. Thus insectivorous species generally nested during the wet season when abundant insects were present: Seed-eating species nested at the start of the dry season when crops were being harvested: Birds of prey nested later still when grass fires provided plenty of cooked prey. This extended breeding of different species overlapping throughout the year meant there was always something to look at.

There was also such infinite variety in the types of nets and their locality. With the idea of attempting a bit of nest photography, I bought an 8 mm cine camera. My first, a Zeiss Movikon, small and compact with an excellent lens, unfortunately had no turret for supplementary lenses; the telephoto lens had to be screwed in place of the standard lens, which made it cumbersome to use and unsuitable for bird photography. I later replaced it with a Canon Zoom–8. Once I had tired of 'zooming' in and out on everything, I found this camera ideal for cine-photography from a hide, where unsightly 'jump-cuts' in the action could be minimised by altering from telephoto to wide-angle between successive shots.

Of course first find your nest. As a child in the Scottish Borders, I became expert at finding bird's nests, but my technique of searching hedgerows by crawling into the centre and looking outwards to see nests silhouetted against the sky could hardly be done in Nigeria where the few hedges were made of a particularly prickly cactus-like euphorbia. Besides, by this period I had put away childish habits, as it did not seem particularly becoming for an adult, particularly a *Bature*, to be seen crawling around in hedgerows.

In fact many smaller Nigerian bird species nested right out in the extremities of the branches of trees as protection against predation by tree snakes. The unusual pendant nests of several species of sunbirds were well camouflaged, looking like untidy bundles of grass. They could generally be found only by patient observation of the parents when building or feeding young; occasionally an aberrant nest would be found hanging conspicuously from a nail under the eave of a building or from an exposed telephone line. The pendant nests made by colonial-nesting weavers, on the other hand, were so conspicuous that little searching was required. Like my old friend the Tailor Bird in India, I discovered the Grey-backed Cameroptera also sewed leaves together.

Many species nested on the ground. Larger birds like plovers, quite easily spotted when sitting on eggs in Scottish fields, were only found in Nigeria with great difficulty by carefully scanning likely bare areas from afar with binoculars. The sitting Senegal Wattled Plover was adept at sneaking off quietly when an intruder was a long way off. Bustards nested in tall grass, laying their cryptically-marked eggs on the bare ground and I only found them by quartering such grassland with Lassie. By contrast, Crowned Cranes, which laid large white eggs on a conspicuous platform of dead grass, also nested in the tall vegetation of paddocks or near swamps and were fairly common around Vom. I was shown some earlier nests by African staff, but later found several after first watching pairs of Crowned Cranes establishing their territories by doing their spectacular dance. Smaller ground-nesting species, Quail Finches, Buntings, Pipits and Finch Larks, built domed or cupped nests often well concealed and usually found only when the birds ran or flew off as one approached.

Like the kingfisher in Britain, the Grey-headed Kingfisher excavated its hole in a bank. Some species, like the Red-throated Bee-eater, preferred safety in numbers and nested in colonies in a roadside cutting. During the prolonged dry season a few species actually nested beneath the ground. The Senegal Hoopoe and the Red-breasted Chat often took over an old dry soak-well or derelict termite mound.

From the window of the isolated Rabies Laboratory I found my first nest. The Senegal Kingfisher, a large and colourful insectivorous bird, became very aggressive when nesting; one once reduced our neighbour's cat to a state of abject misery. A pair took over an old barbet's nest hole in a low tree just outside the laboratory window and jealously guarded their territory. I filmed the bird feeding young at the nest by using a remote release on the camera; the few feet of film I obtained came out sufficiently well to spur me on to greater efforts.

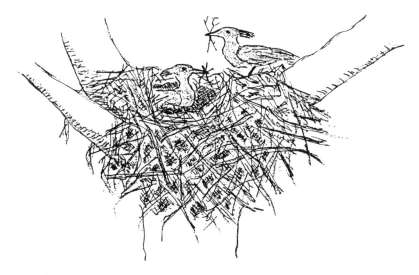

Hammerkops building their nest

Filming by remote control was not very satisfactory, though a lot of my earlier sequences were taken from the car or even a house, using a remote release with the camera on a tripod concealed near the nest. This technique worked reasonably well but was only suitable for short sequences. The ultimate aim was to get lots of film that could be edited ruthlessly to just pick out the best bits. For this a hide was essential.

I experimented with several designs. Prototype hides consisting of sacking draped over sticks and branches were generally too flimsy. In the open flat grassland the conventional cubic hide made of canvas on a frame was far too conspicuous and attracted the curiosity of itinerant farmers, who were not past removing it. To film some species in the grassland I resorted to using a low hide in which I could lie down. My most uncomfortable and spartan one was built into a ditch. Eventually I found that woven grass *Zana* matting, though heavy to carry, was suitable and tended to blend into the landscape very well. Besides, what did we have household staff for but to carry such items? Garden-boy Badung proved his worth on more than one occasion!

My strangest hide, made of sacking on a low frame, was mounted on a one-man inflatable dinghy as used by pilots during the war; a friend on leave, Keith Nixon, managed to buy one for me in an army surplus store and very kindly brought it out by air, though BOAC cabin staff assured him that he would have no need for it on the flight. I spent several hours bobbing around on the Wishi Pool during my last tour, trying to film a pair of grebes at their nest, and as an added bonus captured on film a delightful sequence of young ducklings being led away from this strange floating monstrosity by an adult *Wishi-wishi*.

A number of private tin miners lived on the Plateau, sometimes in total isolation in houses often miles away from anywhere. These houses with their well-manicured gardens were like Vom, little oases in a prairie of grassland. We frequently visited a private miner, Roger Harrison, who married one of the technical officers in the Laboratory, Nesta Scott, tragically killed in a motor accident not long after. They lived for an all too brief period in a delightful old cottage called Kassa some twenty miles south of Vom.

Nearby in a house called Old Kassa lived Kitty Cooke, the first European lady to arrive on the Plateau. Her son, Nigel Cooke, was Senior Resident in Jos during 1961.

The Harrison's house was built into a rocky outcrop – I recall their tiny dining-room had one wall of rock – and their garden was a marvellous wilderness, in which I found, side-by-side, the largest and smallest nests I have ever encountered.

A pair of Hammerkops, crested long-billed brownish birds the size of a domestic fowl, spent weeks carefully arranging a huge pile of sticks and twigs in the low fork of a substantial tree at Kassa. I was astonished to discover that the completed nest was roofed over and more than a metre high. The nest chamber was entered through a small hole in the side, the bird generally landing on the ground, then flying up and

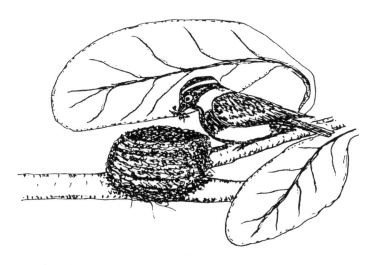

Senegal Puffback Flycatcher building

miraculously disappearing. They were generally so tame that it was possible to observe and film them from a car parked nearby. Old nests, I discovered later, provided very desirable residences for Barn Owls.

It was while sitting in my car one day near the Hammerkop's nest awaiting their return, that I saw on the nearby horizontal branch of a fig tree, a male Senegal Puff-back Flycatcher, a strikingly handsome little black and white bird, building a tiny little cup, five centimetres in diameter, of lichen and cobweb. Later I watched and filmed the female, with quite a bit of chestnut on her, sitting on two eggs.

Glimpses of another species of flycatcher, this time a Pied Flycatcher, in my garden at the start of the 1959 dry season opened new horizons for me. What could I find so intriguing about this little black and white bird? Well, here in its winter haunts south of the Sahara, was a species with which I was familiar in Scotland as a summer visitor, breeding in holes in very old oak trees. There was nothing new about my observation in Vom, as it was well-known that most summer visitors to Europe and Britain spend their winters south of the Sahara. It started me thinking about the possibility of catching and ringing these migrants in their winter haunts.

1959 saw a lot of pre-Independence activity. When Nigeria was first colonised as a Protectorate at the turn of the century, largely to counter the French influence in West Africa and to abolish slavery, the indigenous people were assured it would always be Nigeria for the Nigerians. It was Lugard who instituted a system of indirect rule. It seemed that the early administrators appointed by the Colonial Office found a structure of sorts already in existence. Local Emirs and Chiefs *(Sarki,* pronounced something like 'Sir Ricky') had paramount powers over their subjects, but most required advice on how best to use their powers for the benefit of the whole country. Thus from those early days a system of political advisers of varying ranks was set up. Residents and District Officers jollied the Emirs and Chiefs along and ensured that they kept within certain guidelines laid down by Kaduna, the seat of power and administration. If some Emirs or Chiefs were a trifle more dishonest than others and perhaps siphoned off too much of their revenue for their own personal use, they were replaced if they did not respond to good advice.

Yellow Fever, malaria and the generally unhealthy climate had earned the West Coast of Africa the title *The White Man's Grave.* No good farming highlands, as in East Africa, were available to white settlers who were not allowed freehold title anyway. Whereas during the very early days the expatriates living in the country were mainly government administrators, rapidly the numbers of commercial individuals, like traders, businessmen and miners, built up as more opportunities became available, within certain constraints. For instance even in the 1930s, just before the war, officers in government service were discouraged from taking their wives and families to Nigeria. An efficient vaccine against Yellow Fever and the development of prophylactic anti-malarial drugs during the war were two major factors which made living conditions for Europeans in Nigeria more tolerable.

Before Independence was granted in October 1960, elections were necessary to determine which of several parties would govern. The high rate of illiteracy in the widely dispersed population made it difficult for candidates to address many of their constituents at the village level. So we were treated to the unusual sight of helicopters flying over villages, including Vom on one occasion, dropping large quantities of leaflets bearing the symbol of the party to vote for. In the north the Northern People's Congress (NPC) was the main party and their symbol was three palm trees. The elections were held in December 1959.

Most of the expatriate Laboratory staff considered playing at Electoral Officers beneath their dignity. Reluctant to leave the luxuries of Vom, it was a curt telegram from the Governor General to the acting Director, Tony Thorne, that made us think otherwise.

At very short notice Mike Griffin and I, accompanied by Dantiyi, found ourselves heading south to Shendam just off the Plateau, with a touring kit borrowed from all over Vom station. I placed myself at the disposal of the District Officer, who instructed me to supervise four polling stations nearby in the vicinity of a village called Yelwa. I supervised the setting up of polling booths made of *Zana* grass matting, realising then what superb hides for bird photography could be made from the same material. On polling day the ballot papers only bore symbols, and each person after voting had his wrist indelibly stamped to stop him going to the back of the queue again. In spite of these safeguards, certain irregularities were reported. Political agents for the ruling party stood around prominently.

After voting was finished, I had to escort the lorry with the ballot boxes to Wase. The main town of the Emirate of Wase lay at the foot of the famous Wase Rock, a volcanic trachyte plug 800 feet high which looked like a leaning gate post even from twenty miles away. During my first tour two years previously, I had visited this famous landmark with the family, spending two nights at Pankshin. We were most impressed with the size and vertical profile of this rock with a huge cleft in the centre. A district officer made the first ascent during the late 1950s and a doctor from Jos, Gerry Dunger, subsequently developed several

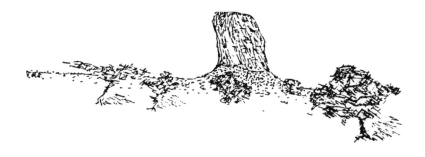

Wase Rock

new routes to the summit. I later learnt from him that a colony of pelicans nested on the flat top in an impregnable position; their nearest feeding place was the Benue River sixty miles away to the south. I think the bee combs, twenty feet long inside the chasm through which one had to ascend, discouraged me more than the dizzy heights from attempting the climb to see the pelican colony.

On this occasion, however, it was after dark when I escorted the lorry to Wase, so I hardly saw the rock, but was aware of its looming presence. After handing over the ballot boxes I returned on my own to my camp bed at Yelwa well after midnight, very nearly having to spend the night in the car when I bogged down in a dry sandy river bed. Unlike my previous excursion to Dengi, no local villagers could be expected to miraculously appear at that time of night. However half an hour of sweaty digging and laying brush under the wheels finally got me out.

The following morning, having the faster car, I conveyed some electoral results from Shendam to Jos, interrupting a cocktail party at the Residency, where I was invited in for a beer. A large tankard of the locally brewed Star beer helped lay the dust, but I felt very embarassed because of my rather dishevelled appearance and fruity odour. In my haste to get to Shendam only two nights previously, I had been unable to borrow a camp bath.

CHAPTER 4

Rinderpest Vaccines
and More Birds

DRONING NORTHWARDS ACROSS THE SAHARA, and unable to sleep on the crowded Boeing 707, I contemplated how fortunate were the children of parents working abroad nowadays. Those expatriates with children at school in Britain were able to fly them out for their school holidays.

In January 1960 a cablegram from home said briefly that Father had died in Moffat as the result of an accident. I was granted compassionate leave and flew back to Scotland for a few days, fortunate to get a seat at such short notice, because it meant travelling on one of BOAC's 'LOLLIPOP SPECIALS', taking children back to school after their Christmas holidays in Nigeria. The plane was packed with kids of all shapes and sizes. The cabin staff had their hands full but coped with an affectionate but firm indulgence. The babel of noise was overwhelming, like a starling roost and drowning the engine noise, as kids compared notes, played up to their peers and showed off – liqueurs with their coffee, indeed!

When Roger was older he would be doing the same. How generous were the present terms of service. We were allowed one extra first-class fare each tour, ostensibly for the mother to go home and see the children, but the money could be used instead to bring the children out for their holidays at economy class rates. The Women's Corona Society provided an admirable service escorting children through Kano, the international airport in the north of Nigeria, and London.

I thought how different it had been in my childhood. In those pre-war years I was boarded in a preparatory school in the south of England from the age of six, while my parents were in India. There was one period when I did not see Dad for nearly five years. Mum only came back once a year during the summer and at her own expense, often sharing a four-berth cabin on a P.&O. Liner with other mothers in the same predicament. For the long summer holidays we would go to different places each year.

The enforced separation from my parents during the six years I was at boarding school made me unhappy at times. I believe I attempted to run away from school once. Mum had put me on the school train as she was soon to catch the liner back to India. There had been the inevitable tearful separation at Victoria station. A few days later, I crept out of the school one evening in the dark, clutching my sixpence pocket-money and remembering to take a clean hankie and was intercepted at the corner shop where I stopped to ask the way to Tilbury Docks, or so the story goes.

At boarding school, Greenways it was called, I was encouraged to take an interest in natural history, as known in those days, and soon could identify the birds found nearby. This enthusiasm for studying wild-life did not seem to be detrimental to my schooling, though one school report commented; *'We wish that he would put into his work the same energy he displays over anything connected with birds . . .'*

In spite of my hurried departure from Vom, I was too late to see my father laid to rest, only arriving late on the day of the funeral. However I remained in Moffat about a month, and left his affairs in the hands of the family solicitor. Back in Vom, where June and Roger remained during my absence, I soon got back into vaccine production.

By this time the new Tissue-cultured Rinderpest Vaccine (TCRV) was ready for field trials. The pioneer work of attenuating Rinderpest virus in tissue culture was carried out in Kenya by Plowright & Ferris, though their work on the use of this attenuated virus as a vaccine was not published until 1962. But by 1960 it was obvious that another vaccine, and it looked as if TCRV might fill this need, was urgently required for use in the field in West Africa to replace the fragile LRV. An internationally-funded rinderpest eradication scheme (JP15) was due to start in the north of Nigeria and adjacent countries in 1962. Financial aid was provided by USAID and the EEC for this campaign.

My boss, guide and mentor in the Virology Division, 'Johnny' Johnson, had obtained the tissue-cultured attenuated virus from Plowright in 1959 and made a seed stock, from which vaccine batches were made. Using local materials, Johnny had then built up stocks of vaccine which urgently required testing in the field. I inadvertently became involved on the fringe of the sort of situation which plagues rivals in the same field of research, for it so happened that Johnny's findings were published before those of the eminent Plowright. More dreadful still was the fact that Plowright learnt of Johnny's published work through some obscure West Indian magazine.

I thought it all very funny at the time and was sufficiently new to the game not to take it too seriously, but just got on with my contribution to the overall grand scheme. The vaccine virus was grown in cell cultures prepared from calf kidneys, but few young calves could be spared from the farm. It soon became necessary to use kidneys obtained from bovine foetuses which were available at the slaughter-slab in Jos, sixteen miles away.

It became one of my duties to go early in the morning and get them. Situated near the market, the slaughter-slab was a large unroofed concrete area, divided by deep gutters down which blood and waste flowed into a sump, and surrounded by a low parapet on which rows of hooded vultures usually sat, awaiting the choice bits that oozed down the gutters, or glided low overhead to join their companions on the other side. Hygiene was at a minimum, as blood and gore lay everywhere around the carcases. Some attempt was made to keep the carcases fairly clean by laying the meat on the flayed and spread out skins.

The poor beasts were killed according to the dictates of Mohammedanism by having their throats cut while cast on the concrete floor and roped to prevent too much struggling. Invariably there were a few healthy pregnant cows amongst the animals slaughtered most weekdays, and the whole uterus was usually discarded as offal, that is until the

Sarkin Pawa, the head butcher, realised from our interest in them that the foetuses offered some financial return.

Hausa love to haggle and get great enjoyment from bargaining. I found myself at considerable disadvantage bargaining with the assistance of one of the laboratory technicians for a suitable uterus. To ensure sterility, it was necessary to get the foetus still enclosed in the uterus and as clean as possible.

The haggling was often negotiated with much shouting across the width of the slaughter-slab, the *Sarkin Pawa* holding up a uterus over the gutter, quite prepared to drop it in the filth if the offered price was not to his liking. I could only judge the size of the foetus by the overall size of the uterus and the ease with which the big fellow held it up, so tended to be over generous with my offer.

Having secured a trophy, I then raced back to Vom and we would process the kidneys from the foetus. In a sterile environment, a room specially set aside for such processing and previously sterilised by ultra-violet lights over the bench, the foetal kidneys were removed, chopped into tiny pieces and digested with enzymes using a magnetic stirrer. I was constantly amused by the way visitors, even government ministers, looking in through one of the side windows of the sterile room, were always fascinated by the way the little magnet rotated apparently of its own volition.

The strained and coarsely-filtered cell suspension was centrifuged and the cells resuspended in an enriched growth medium in large flat-sided glass flasks. With a modicum of good luck, which made me wonder at times whether we should mumble an incantation or two over the brew, the cells grew on the glass to form a monolayer, which could then be infected with the TCRV virus.

When faced with something beyond her comprehension, my mother-in-law used to say, 'It's the way you hold your mouth, Vic,' but the explanation for success with tissue cultures was much more based on scientific reasoning. The glassware and equipment used had to be spotlessly clean and the reagents and medium made with the purest ingredients. The cells of each batch had to be carefully monitored and some always retained uninfected with the TCRV virus to ensure there were no latent viruses from the original foetus. Cells could be passaged a limited number of times by digesting them off the glass with enzymes and splitting into another two or three flasks.

Cells could also be stored indefinitely at ultra-low temperatures, provided they were frozen slowly in a sort of anti-freeze mixture and we first relied on a weekly delivery of dry ice from Kano which kept our improvised insulated cabinet at the required temperature of −70°C. Our biggest problem was guaranteeing the regular supply of dry ice, until we acquired a Verikold ultra-low-temperature deep freeze. Thus one calf or foetus offered the potential for theoretically providing sufficient mono-layers to produce many thousands of doses of vaccine, an important ethical factor when considering the number of goats or rabbits we had to use to produce other rinderpest vaccines.

The first trial batches of TCRV showed great promise when tested in a few of the laboratory cattle, but it was necessary to carry out more extensive field trials. What better place to perform them than in the regions where the new vaccine would be used.

In 1960, not long after my return from Scotland, Dantiyi and I found ourselves down in the Western Region of Nigeria at a government farm in Fashola near Ilorin, where I completed the first field trial in N'dama cattle, a breed which was highly susceptible to rinderpest and in which LRV was normally used.

To evaluate any new vaccine it is necessary to show it is fairly tough and able to withstand normal field conditions, then prove its safety in the animals in which it will be used, its potency, its immunogenicity and later the duration of the immunity it confers.

The cattle at Fashola had received different doses of trial production batches of the new TCRV. They were examined daily and none showed any adverse reaction.

A fortnight later the vaccinated animals were challenged, that is inoculated with DGV. All survived without any reaction. The unfortu-nate unvaccinated control N'dama cattle which were also challenged, became highly fevered and very sick and those that did not die were later killed. With a dearth of fresh meat at Fashola, I tried some steaks from one of these fevered animals after carefully performing an autopsy on it. I found the steaks deliciously tender, thus confirming in my own mind a fact that was generally well known amongst the field veterinary staff. Rinderpest-infected animals provided good meat because the fever tenderised the meat by breaking down the fibres.

I returned to Vom by air with the results of the first successful field trial, to find that Johnny had already left for the Eastern Region of Nigeria to start a similar trial using dwarf Muturu cattle at a government farm called Ezamgbo near Abakaliki. With hardly a break in Vom I hastened down by road, this time taking June and Roger, and arrived there to find that the situation had deteriorated into something approaching a ludicrous comic opera.

The Chief Veterinary Officer in Eastern Nigeria, an Ibo named Mbaeliachi — dare I say he was rather irreverently called 'Bellyache' behind his back — agreed to some of the cattle at Ezamgbo being used in a highly irregular manner, however, he bought Muturu cattle from neighbouring villages. Without holding them for a period in quarantine, they were introduced directly to the farm where most of the thousand Muturu cattle were in a susceptible state. Unknown to him, rinderpest was smouldering in the neighbourhood. Thus the stage was set.

Johnny vaccinated the animals selected for the trial not knowing that some of the recently introduced animals were incubating the disease. When these showed symptoms of rinderpest soon after, the vaccine, of course, immediately came under suspicion, even though there had been no adverse affects at Fashola.

Once rinderpest was confirmed, Mbaeliachi, to his great and eternal credit, admitted cattle had been introduced from outside. The entire herd at Ezamgbo was at risk from rinderpest. After urgent telephone consultations between our Director, Tony Thorne, and Mbaeliachi, the situation was turned to our advantage. It was agreed there was nothing to lose by vaccinating the entire herd at Ezamgbo with the new TCRV. It was emphasised any cattle incubating rinderpest would die. As it was the overall mortality was negligible and the new vaccine came out an outright winner.

We spent a few days in Abakaliki Catering Rest House while I visited some of the markets on patrol looking for further cases of rinderpest. One market EKE IMOHA, where we found some cases, was picturesquely set in tall forest but very primitive. Many of the native stall-holders were decorated with yellow ochre and I was fascinated to see that some played freely with green snakes, draping them around their

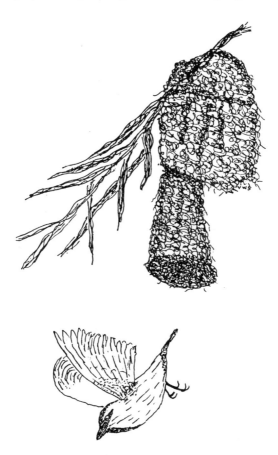

Spectacled Weaver leaving nest

necks – I did not approach close enough to determine whether they were harmless tree snakes or highly venomous green mambas.

Amongst the trees on the periphery of the market I was saddened to see a group of emaciated horses from the north, all old in the tooth, awaiting their fate with resignation. I had heard it was customary for wealthy Ibos to beat a horse to death as a sort of ritual sacrifice, to indicate what a 'Big' man the beater was. I was glad to get back to Vom.

Nigeria was granted Independence on October 31st, 1960, as a prelude to becoming a Republic within the Commonwealth on October 1st 1963. The Independence Declaration was read in many places all over the country, in English by the Senior Resident and in the native dialects by the local chief. In Vom there were modest celebrations. Dr Taylor read his bit and the local *Sarkin Vom* read the message in Hausa. Dr Taylor, the Director of Veterinary Research, having fulfilled his contract to see the Federal Veterinary Services into independence, left soon after as did several other senior staff.

There was at this time a scarcity of adequately-trained Nigerian professional staff, so expatriates were encouraged to remain. Those remaining in the permanent expatriate staff had to decide whether they wanted to stay on and for how long. Up to this period, we had been members of the Colonial Service, administered by the Colonial Office, but the connotation 'Colonial' now became a dirty word, so staff who remained became members of the Overseas Civil Service, attached to the Commonwealth Office, until it later merged into the Foreign Office. Later still it became the Ministry of Overseas Development (MOD), under British Labour Government, or synonymously the Overseas Development Administration (ODA), under Conservative Government, to the confusion of poor pensioners like me who were never quite sure to whom we should address our queries.

A Lump Sum Compensation Scheme (LSCS – 'Lumpers') was introduced for the benefit of those expatriate staff who would lose their careers and pension entitlements, or who preferred not to continue once self-government was introduced. It is notable that the incoming Nigerian Government agreed to continue the Pension Scheme which had been in operation and this they still continue to do long after Independence. The inevitable forms for registering for 'Lumpers' had to be completed.

Factors were calculated on age and service, to encourage staff to stay on during the transitional period until trained Nigerians were ready to take over. At Independence, there were very few qualified Nigerian veterinary surgeons, though several were training overseas. After some deliberation, and with much discussion with others in the same boat I elected to stay on for another six years, by which time I would be forty and my factor at its peak.

This meant that we had to give the matter of Roger's schooling some serious thought, because he would then be ten. We had little option but to consider sending Roger back to a school in Britain, though the new Capital school in Kaduna had recently started to take the children of senior civil servants. My old school Greenways had been evacuated from Bognor Regis during the early months of the war to Wiltshire and had remained there. On making a few inquiries I was pleased to learn that they would take Roger as a boarder when he was seven, so I planned my tours to allow us to be on leave at that time. In the meantime a day school in Bukuru catered for children of pre-school age.

Marie Prescott, whose husband Bernard worked in NESCO, ran a small day school on the outskirts of Bukuru, to which Roger and many of his contemporary playmates were taken every morning about the time we breakfasted. All parents were rostered weekly for the 'school bus' and when my turn came every two or three weeks I would collect half a dozen children in my car, deposit them at school, then hurry back for a hasty breakfast. They had to be collected from school about the time we stopped for lunch.

About this time I can recall Sunday visits to see progress on the Bornu Extension Railway to Maiduguri. By 1960 work had proceeded some distance along the track from a point off the main line south of Jos. When the plans were submitted, I believe a diversion became necessary to take the line through Tafawa Balewa, the Prime Minister's home town, and install a station there, which added considerably to the costs of construction. Returning for my second tour on M. V. *Accra*, we had met a couple, Dick and Ann Keays, with a daughter about Roger's age. For a while they lived in Bukuru and Dick was the medical officer for the engineering company which was laying the line. On several Sundays we went out along the track with him to visit his clinics, suitably impressed with the progress on each subsequent visit. Also there were different birds to see in the Guinea Savanna, or Orchard Bush as it was called, through which the line progressed once it left the Plateau.

All these activities so soon after my return from Scotland, made me put aside thoughts of migrant birds and birds' nests. It was not until the 1960 wet season that I met Bob Sharland, an accountant from Kano, who already was catching and ringing birds in Northern Nigeria, using mist-nets and rings supplied by the British Trust for Ornithology (BTO), bearing the return address *British Museum, London*. Later he started the Nigerian scheme, using rings which bore the return address *Museum, Jos, Nigeria*. Bob sold me some mist-nets and supplied me with a few rings.

Mist-nets, of fine nylon like fishnet stockings, were made in several sizes. Nets about 7 to 10 metres long and 2 metres high were suitable for use in my garden. Woven lengthwise were stouter lengths of very strong braided nylon, called shelf strings, which were supposed to be attached to poles at either end. At first I had to improvise, as wooden poles were unavailable and I had to resort to ten foot lengths of gas or water piping, borrowed from the PWD, and very heavy and inconvenient to carry. In my garden, however, I found the nets could quite simply be secured to trees with fencing wire. The net hung quite loosely between these tight shelf strings so birds hitting the net would lie uninjured in a pocket over them.

Used for many years in Japan to catch birds to eat, their value for catching birds for research studies was realised after the war. They are an invaluable tool. Undeterred by my first unsuccessful efforts to net snipe – like trying to catch minnows in a dam with a tea strainer – I next put up nets amongst the bushes in my garden, shaded by colourful Poinsettia, Jacaranda and Poinciana, the splendid Flame of the Forest. I was rewarded with success almost immediately. I expected Pied Fly-catchers which I already knew were present, but was pleasantly surprised also to net Garden Warblers as they passed through in considerable numbers on their way to the more forested areas further south.

Mist nets are renowned for catching the more secretive species not normally sighted, and in later years I caught (and photographed) an Ortolan Bunting, not listed in Bannerman's Bible, and demonstrated marked seasonal movements, one way but not the other, of several migrant species, like the Icterine Warbler and the Spotted Flycatcher, which nest in Europe or Britain and spend their non-breeding period very sensibly in warmer climes south of the Sahara, some only passing through Nigeria on their way further south.

This was an auspicious start indeed. Little was known about the movements of these birds, because they skulked in dense foliage. I caught the Garden Warblers in nets sited deep in shrubbery, some as early as September. Bannerman only listed sight records from November on-wards, so I felt the world should know about my findings. I wrote to *Ibis*, the Journal of the British Ornithologist's Union (BOU).

The Editor of *Ibis* at that time, Dr James Monk, accepted my short note and helpfully polished it up suitable for publication. Later, when I visited him on leave, we discussed whether I should weigh any migrants I caught. About this time other workers had learnt that long distance migrants put on considerable weight in the form of body fat, which they metabolised to provide the energy required for flying long distances across water or inhospitable country like the Sahara Desert. This abundant body fat explained why the Romans liked these tasty morsels – they were like butter-balls. Even in those days countless birds on their migration south through Italy were caught with birdlime and slaughtered for the table to feed a society which was becoming increasingly decadent.

I first borrowed a cumbersome triple-beam balance from the

Laboratory, but later purchased a set of Pesola spring balances. Weighing birds in Nigeria in autumn after completion of their southbound journey across the Sahara provided information on their arrival weights, very low because the birds had utilised most of their reserves. The much heavier weights of birds in spring before their northward journey later allowed for some interesting comparisons.

One Pied Flycatcher, which arrived exhausted, spent the entire season in my garden and made an important contribution to science. I was fortunate enough to retrap it no less than five times; this tiny bird obviously found our garden to its liking because it put on an astonishing 74% of its autumn arrival weight before heading north in the spring.

Nets were erected in the garden almost all the time during the spring and autumn passages, but nearly all the bird movements occurred early in the morning or in the hour before dusk. At night fruit bats, particularly around the mango tree, got themselves inextricably caught but since we were surveying all wild animals for rabies, I killed them painlessly before extricating them, rather that run the gauntlet of their sharp teeth.

Each morning before going to work at 7.00 a.m., I would check the nets and ring any birds. At breakfast time, school bus roster permitting, I would ring any others removed by June. Generally by breakfast time the *Harmattan* was sufficiently strong to disturb the nets, and the sun high enough to make the nets obvious. Local birds were not deterred from making our garden their home and once they learnt the position of the nets they tended to avoid them, though several 'slow-learners' were caught repeatedly.

'A bird in the hand is worth two in the bush'. By netting them I was able to positively identify in the hand a number of the local garden species. Not possessing a camera for still photography, June and I took slow-motion cine-film of several of the more colourful species as they were released from the hand. I was astonished to find that many birds remained in the hand for a second or two on their backs when released. The home movies produced some startling results, like a series of disjointed conjuring tricks, but showed the birds well and their exquisite colours.

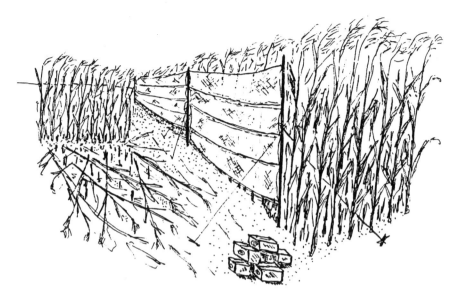

Mist nets in sugar cane

And how exquisite or curious some of the birds were. A tiny Malachite Kingfisher, brilliant ultramarine and rufous, which I caught at Ouree Dam on one of our earlier netting excursions outside Vom, lay indignantly on its back on my hand, squinting at the end of its bill, greenish-blue crest erect and falling forward. One European Wryneck, with beautiful vermiculated grey-brown plumage, turned its head almost through a full circle.

Honey-Guides were unusual in that they trembled in the hand. The very fine tremor became most apparent after half a minute or so, as if holding a vibrator. I netted several Black-throated Honey-Guides and they all behaved in this curious manner. Only once did I hear their excited chattering call in the garden, when bees occupied our chimney.

Bees abounded around Vom and their numbers were reflected by the numerous colourful bee-eaters of several species seen in the vicinity. Carmine, Red-throated, White-throated, Little and occasionally Swallow-tailed Bee-eaters appeared at different times of the year.

Although they feed on other insects, the bee-eaters' main prey, bees, proved to be a serious menace, especially when they built their nests in the most improbable places. At the farm, for instance, some of the gate-posts were made of wide hollow metal pipes with holes for bolting on the hinges. Bee swarms sometimes mistook these pipes for hollow logs. A swarm occupied one such hollow metal gate-post and severely stung the farm manager, Murray Denoon, when he allowed the gate to slam shut. The bees normally nested in hollow trees, which were rather scarce around Vom, so they frequently took over crevices in rocks or occasionally nested under the ground in old termite mounds.

However in Vom itself the swarms occupied chimneys or settled under the eaves of houses and laboratory buildings. The eaves of the newer buildings were all boxed in, but often the bees found the merest crevice or hole. Where such nests were close to habitation and posed a threat, their removal necessitated the services of the P.W.D.'Bees-man' who worked at night when the bees were at home. He would spray with what he called 'Cuppentile' – white spirits or turpentine – which seemed to stupefy the bees. Then sometimes he would burn the hive and strip out the combs of honey. The next morning one would notice gaping holes under the eaves, and he would sell the combs, not a very appetising sight when viewed in a bucket as the combs and honey were generously mixed with bee larvae, overall perfused with an odour of resin.

Vicious these African Killer bees were indeed and many the tales we heard of their very aggressive behaviour, especially when they swarmed during the humid weather at the start of the wet season. Animals, like a pagan pony called Mandy which we looked after for a short while, were stung to death – in her case she disturbed a swarm which had settled in her food box.

Humans on occasion were severely threatened and several friends had nasty frights. A few years after we left Nigeria we read in our local Western Australian press of a climbing instructor who was stung to death

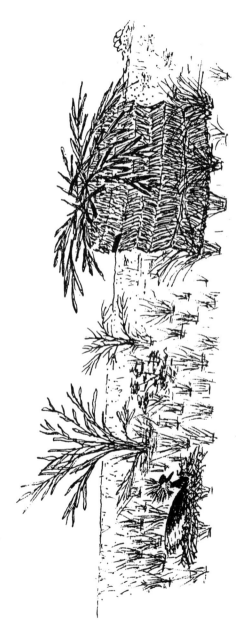

Crowned Crane's nest and hide

while taking a party up Wase Rock, where honeycombs twenty feet long had been reported in some of the crevices. The Army took six days to recover the body, in the process causing so much disturbance and using so much insecticide that the pelicans abandoned their nest site on top for a year or two.

Our moment of truth occurred when I shot a rabid dog on the far side of Vom early during our last wet season. I delivered the corpse to the rabies laboratory for examination and after lunch I asked Badung to mop up spilt blood in the car boot. He sponged out the boot with Dettol and something in the smell aroused the bees in our chimney. They had been acting a bit temperamentally because of the humid weather. Badung was lucky to make it to the house with only a sting or two. For the rest of the afternoon June and I, Lassie, Dantiyi and Badung were confined to the house by angry bees which hurtled around the windows. After dark we escaped and later found three of our four free-range White Leghorn hens stung to death. On the comb of one I counted over a hundred stings The one survivor had escaped in long grass. Our cat, Pyewacket, had also found refuge somewhere and was untouched. How on earth did our cat get called by such an unusual name?

CHAPTER 5

Pets, Rabies,
other Animals, and Owls

PLATEAU PLAYERS PUT ON AN AMATEUR PRODUCTION of the play *Bell, Book and Candle* soon after we returned to Vom for my second tour. In this play about a modern day witch, a cat called Pyewacket helped in the casting of spells. What an unusual name we thought, so our fourth Nigerian kitten became Pyewacket, to the consternation of kind friends who later looked after her when we were on leave.

Sadly two previous kittens met with untimely ends. Number one had the temerity to approach Lassie when she was having her supper. Number two escaped from my car when I stopped at a fallen tree across the road on my way to Lagos. A third, Sputnik (no prize for guessing why), brought down to Lagos by June in a BOAC flightbag, remained there with the Slaters at the end of our first tour.

While she was still very young, I spayed Pyewacket on our dining-room table, Nurse June assisting, using instruments borrowed from the veterinary clinic. She turned into a very placid and affectionate cat, a tabby with the traditional wild-cat markings and long droopy whiskers. Her long-haired coat required regular grooming and suggested she had Persian blood in her. During the dry season her thick pelt rarely seemed to cause her heat stress, but provided an endless source of entertainment.

When the *Harmattan* blew at its worst, the intense dryness of the air caused a considerable build up of static electricity which, for instance, frequently gave us shocks from car doors. Hair crackled when combed. At this time of year my favourite party trick was to stroke Pyewacket, then let her smell my finger. A visible spark seemed to jump from finger to nose, invariably making her recoil and blink her eyes. She must have got a kick out of it for she always came back for more.

Liking her home comforts, she slept on our bed most nights. If she wanted to go out during the night, she became adept at rolling off under the mosquito net without displacing it too much. She could climb back on the bed under the net equally proficiently. This was an improvement on our second kitten, Tinkerbell. When still very young, she found the top of our mosquito net made an ideal hammock, though her efforts to go to bed did nothing for the net itself.

One night on returning from her nightly perambulation, Pyewacket brought with her onto the bed a trophy which she introduced to us. From the little 'Prrp, Prrp' noises she was making, like a cat calling her kittens when offering them something, we should have realised something was afoot. We were not at all amused with the live musk shrew she released on the bed. In the evacuation in the dark, Lassie, who slept at our bedside, got trodden on adding to the general pandemonium. The shrew somehow escaped, leaving behind a sickly-sweet musky smell, which was supposed to deter predators but obviously had been no deterrent to Pyewacket.

Of small animals we encountered very few. An African Hedgehog appeared in our garden on one occasion. Lassie's barking drew our attention to it, but she found it just as prickly as those she had encountered in England.

At the beginning of the first dry season in our new house, Dantiyi found a dormouse in the empty bath where he washed our clothes. He brought it to me and I identified it as the Small Dormouse, a common savanna species, distinct from the Large Dormouse which lived in the forest. We thought it had been feeding in the guava tree by the bathroom window, so I let it go outside, much regretting my generous impulse later.

The social highlight of the year, the Caledonian Ball, a splendid dress affair full of pageantry, was due a few weeks later in November. It was one of those rare occasions during the year when I dressed up in a dinner suit, not having traditional Scottish dress as my knobbly knees did not do justice to a kilt. Eager to try the new dinner suit I had bought during my previous leave, I was taken aback when June told me she had found a dormouse's nest containing four hairless babies built in the armpit. Furthermore the sleeve was hanging by mere threads because mother dormouse had used the lining to make the nest very cosy, so the suit was totally ruined. I had to struggle into Father's old one. My Insurance Company refused the claim, drawing attention to the small print which specified that vermin damage was not covered. I thought how heartless could they be to call such appealing creatures vermin.

Many Scots worked in and around Jos. As a result the Plateau Caledonian Society was a flourishing concern and held three functions each year. On Burns Night, there was the inevitable supper at which the traditional delicacy of the Scots, haggis, was eaten with all the trimmings and due reverence and ceremony, washed down with drams of whisky or that Elixir-of-the-Gods Athol Brose, and accompanied by much of the Bard's poetry. Mid-year there was the Chief's Night, a sort of social gathering of the clans. On or near St Andrew's day in November the occasion of the year, the Caledonian Ball, was held.

We were always warned a function was drawing nigh when we heard strange gurgling, squealing noises from just down the road beyond our bungalow, where piper Arnold MacLeod lived. It seemed that the dry atmosphere on the Plateau did queer things to his bagpipes, I believe necessitating the use of treacle, or was it honey, to soften the leather. It always took him a wee while to get the concoction out of the bag.

With the name Smith and born in India, the Committee were only convinced I was eligible to join the Caledonian Society, when I produced evidence of my father's birthplace at a farm called Dalfibble, near Dumfries, to prove I had Scottish blood in my veins.

I often questioned what right did we have to criticise the Africans for their rigid tribalism when the Caledonian Society provided such tangible proof of our tribal customs. One memorable occasion at Jos Airport was intended to provide some publicity for BOAC, though I wondered what the Africans at the airport made of the spectacle of a haggis on a silver

platter, escorted by a number of gentlemen dressed in kilts, being piped
with due ceremony off the plane.

Nigeria was so heavily populated with people there seemed little room
for wild game animals which were such a feature of the east African
scene. Few wild animals could be found around Vom, though the
occasional duiker was relentlessly pursued by the Africans if this small
species of antelope dared show itself.

A tragic episode happened soon after we arrived in Vom. An Agricultural Officer at Riyom Poultry Farm was badly mauled by a leopard
not many miles from Vom. When local Fulani complained they were
losing calves, Brian very bravely but rather foolishly crawled in amongst
rocks where the leopard had cubs. He took with him his shotgun in a
dangerous state of disrepair, which I believe misfired. The female leopard
swiped him across the face. Very lucky he was indeed to survive the
dreadful wounds which resulted in facial paralysis.

Undeterred by this event some friends of ours, Gill and Geoff Strong
of one of the local mining companies, reared a leopard cub, though
good sense prevailed in the end and it was eventually donated to the
Zoo in Jos because of its unpredictable behaviour when it grew up.

This was also the fate of a cheetah called Mai Lafiya, reared by the
Godfreys on the staff of the West African Institute for Trypanosomiasis
Research (WAITR), who also reared orphan chimpanzees and once a
baby baboon. Mai Lafiya, a beautiful and gentle animal, had the run of
their house and garden and was only chained on a running lead when
the family were away. Once calling at their house in their absence I
found Mai Lafiya badly tangled in his chain, which was wrapped tight
round his hock, with the spring-clip gripping his Achilles tendon. Unable
to release the chain without using pliers and some force, thereby causing
him considerable pain but no lasting damage, I was astonished that he
only lay on his side and purred loudly as I freed him. Kept as a family
pet, he behaved well with the children, became very domesticated and

accompanied the family on walks. Alas, he took to playfully chasing the laboratory sheep. No doubt he thought that a great game, but the poor sheep were soon reduced to a state of abject terror.

Leopard and cheetah were donated to Jos Zoo, part of a Cultural Centre, the brain child of Bernard Fagg, the first Director. Within the complex there was a Museum, containing strange relics of a cultured past, like the Ife bronzes and the Nok Pottery heads. There was also an eating place, called very appropriately THE BITE OF BENIN where native dishes like groundnut curry, palm oil chop and other traditional African foods were served.

We often took visitors to this interesting place and the Zoo was a great attraction with children. Most of the enclosures and cages were small but nicely landscaped. Amongst the several local species of animals kept in cages, some were tame enough to handle. The keepers were always eager to bring some of them out, particularly the smaller monkeys, and let children fondle them. Visitors often asked what strange creature lay behind the sign ZUKIPAS ONLY.

The baby chimps earlier reared by the Godfreys and other expatriate staff at WAITR were all acquired as orphans from the Cameroons. Tragically their mothers had been shot by hunters and to discourage this deplorable market, WAITR stopped taking them, once it was realised that they might be fostering the demand. Those that were reared, however, were treated as members of the family, and later became members of the staff in WAITR, each with his own personal file. They contributed in a minor way to the advancement of knowledge about sleeping sickness by participating in chemotherapy trials, and some could even take their own rectal temperatures. When a drop of blood for a blood film was required from them, they would reluctantly hold out their finger and whimper a little with eyes screwed tight, just like a young child. A piece of fruit as a reward soon had them smiling again.

In the vicinity of Vom carnivorous nocturnal hunters like mongooses, civet cats and genets occasionally broke into chicken runs and created havoc. A major disaster occurred at the EPU one night when some wild animal broke into the broiler section and killed several broilers by nipping their necks. However, many others were suffocated as the panic caused a monumental pile-up in one corner.

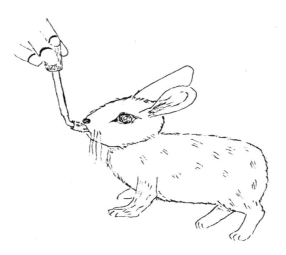

Leveret feeding

On one occasion fertile eggs surplus to our requirements in the laboratory were inadvertently allowed to hatch and I took a few of the day-old chicks home. We tended them till they came into lay but, alas, not for long. The wire-bottomed chicken house in which they roosted behind our bungalow was no deterrent to a hungry beast. We never discovered what left the pathetic carcases lying around the garden.

A young Black-bellied Bustard given to us as a newly-hatched chick also suffered the same fate. It was harder to bear the loss of that family pet, which enjoyed accompanying us on walks through long grass feeding on any grasshoppers we disturbed. It was four months old and fully grown when killed. About the same time we found a leveret, a young hare, in the grass behind the house and the two became inseparable in the garden during the day. Fortunately Hoppy was kept in an old rabbit cage on the back verandah at night, so survived a bit longer.

Dantiyi and other household servants must have thought us all a trifle eccentric wanting to keep such wild animals as pets, when to them they were just a source of food. Even dogs were considered a great delicacy by some of the tribal groups and in Vom Village some were reared purely for eating. The breeding bitches were never in very good shape. Thin with pendulous dugs they grabbed what scraps they could find. When they were nursing puppies, however, they were always thrown a bit more, and the puppies at weaning were invariably as fat as butter-balls.

With many dogs around, Rabies was always a problem. I recall being told that each year several cases were reported in humans at Vom Mission Hospital, but quite a few went undiagnosed or unconfirmed, because of the lack of laboratory facilities.

Soon after I arrived in Vom, and while on some other business, I visited Vom Mission Hospital and was allowed to look into one of their isolation huts, a sparsely furnished tiny room in which there was a raised bed, little more than an earthen platform. Lying on it, on a grass mat, was a young pagan child, who had been bitten on the leg by a dog some weeks previously. She had had no treatment at the time. The wound had healed, but she had scratched the site raw and been brought in demented. When I saw her she was not violent, much the opposite; perhaps she was sedated. I remember her lying there with an expression of anxiety, apprehensive, her eyes never still. She died soon after in convulsions. Rabies was put down as the cause of death.

There, but for the grace of God (and a vigilant father), go I, for when I think of Rabies I am reminded of an episode from my remote childhood when we lived in Delhi. Buster, one of the Cocker Spaniel pups and my favourite, reappeared after an absence of a few days and was seen entering my bedroom which had a door opening onto the verandah. Woken from my afternoon snooze by the dog on my bed, and on the point of putting my hand out to touch the dog, I recall Dad suddenly entering through the inside door, carrying his shotgun, with a strange expression on his face. It was many years later that I learnt Buster had died of Rabies and of the dreadful quandary Dad had been faced with. Shooting Buster on my bed might have inflicted an indelible trauma on me. As it was, he managed to hook the barrel of the shotgun through Buster's collar and swing him outside.

During my time in Nigeria pet dogs and cats were vaccinated with the Flury vaccine repeated every year, which gave good protection. Some cases of suspected vaccination breakdown were reported, but they were difficult to investigate. I remember a veterinary officer recounting an incident he had witnessed on tour. While he watched, a newly-qualified veterinary assistant, eager to impress his superior, had carefully boiled the syringe, then sucked up near-boiling water from the saucepan into the syringe to reconstitute the vaccine.

The control of Rabies also depended on periodically thinning out the obvious stray dogs. The main threat came from the mangy ownerless curs which seemed to appear from nowhere, but particularly at the beginning of the wet season. Much as I disliked doing it, I was always ready to shoot any strange stray dogs seen around the residential parts of Vom, especially if they were acting a bit oddly. Any pets, whether vaccinated or not, which had contact with such animals were impounded in the Rabies Kennel at Vom Veterinary Clinic and kept under observation for a month, as were any animals which bit people, particularly children.

Rabies Kennels were an integral part of any Veterinary Clinic, even in remote areas. The clinician could observe a dog, which may have bitten a human or another animal or showed signs suspicious of Rabies, without exposing himself to any risk. At that time the World Health Organisation recommended that, if such an animal was still alive and healthy a week later, it could be considered non-infectious at the time of the bite and released. Thus any contact animals could not have become infected. If a human had been bitten and had started a course of vaccine injections, as many as twenty-six with the old Pasteur vaccine, they could be discontinued.

Dogs in the early stages of Rabies went off their food, so any which were impounded were always offered food and water. Unlike the disease in humans, where the swallowing reflex becomes so painful it causes fear of water, hence Hydrophobia, in dogs this was not a constant symptom. A change of temperament, apprehension, bizarre behaviour like 'fly-catching' were often the first signs noticed by the owner. After a short 'furious' stage when rabid dogs could be violent, they usually lapsed into the 'dumb' stage, with mouth hanging open drooling saliva and looking as if they had a foreign body lodged in the throat, by which time the dogs were also showing signs of paralysis. Beware 'the-bone-in-the-throat' syndrome was good advice given to new chums, for even

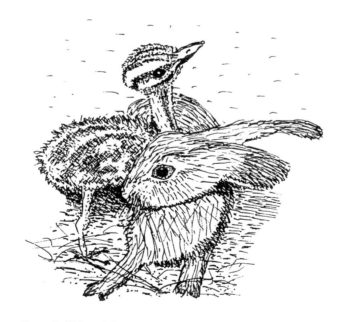

Bustard chick and Leveret

veterinary surgeons were known to put their bare hands down the throat looking for a non-existent bone.

Cats were as susceptible to rabies as dogs and were vaccinated with half a dog dose. Cases in cats were less frequent, the assumption being that they kept out of the way of rabid dogs. Nevertheless I recall three cats which were badly bitten on the face and each died of rabies within three weeks. All were suckling kittens and presumably stood their ground in front of a rabid dog and paid the penalty. It is unlikely that rabid dogs would be deterred by a cat facing up to them. Cats showed much the same symptoms as dogs, yet a relatively common injury in cats, a broken lower jaw sustained by falling off a verandah onto a concrete surface, was often misdiagnosed, such was the reluctance to examine physically the mouth of any animal with Rabies-like symptoms. When the Veterinary Clinic acquired an X-ray machine, such injuries were diagnosed correctly.

All warm-blooded animals can become infected with rabies and cases in cattle, horses, sheep, goats and pig were confirmed in Vom. In West Africa the dog was the main carrier of the disease, as in parts of Asia. Wild animals, like jackals, arctic and red foxes or vampire bats, posed no problem in Nigeria because they did not occur there or were very scarce. Nevertheless the few wild animal carcases submitted to the laboratory were examined diligently.

Rabies was sometimes misdiagnosed in grazing animals, which were considered 'dead-end' hosts, unlikely to bite other animals. I recall one Fulani cow which was treated for three days for hypomagnesaemia, lowered magnesium levels in the blood causing a condition called Grass Staggers, before Rabies was correctly diagnosed.

If a human was bitten by a stray dog which was subsequently killed, the carcase was always sent to the Rabies Laboratory for examination. I was never very pleased if a dead dog or two arrived on a Saturday morning, as they sometimes did, when thoughts were already turning to a beer in the club. The examination took some time and involved cutting out the brain by sawing open the skull with a hand saw, wearing suitable protective clothing, an apron, heavy gloves and a face mask.

Smears made from various parts of the brain were stained by a rapid Sellar's stain and examined under the microscope for characteristic Negri Bodies which were frequently but not always seen in the fully developed disease. The first report either stated 'Negri bodies seen – positive for rabies' or 'No Negri bodies seen – results of biological tests to follow.'

The biological test confirmed the diagnosis. Portions of brain tissue were homogenised in a mortar with antibiotic solution, centrifuged and the supernatant inoculated into anaesthetised white mice which were generally killed by the virus within three weeks if the tissue was positive. It seemed a brutal method of making a diagnosis, yet essential for safeguarding human life. At that time the current belief that Rabies was inevitably fatal to humans once clinical signs developed, sufficiently justified the use of mice to diagnose the disease.

Later an immunofluorescence test was used on brain smears. This was considered more reliable, yet still not one hundred per cent accurate. The accuracy of diagnostic tests depended on the degree of specificity of the reagents and earlier ones caused some problems with diagnosis. For instance, a virus isolated in Lagos from fruit bats and known as Lagos Bat Virus, was originally thought to be different from Rabies, yet many years after I left Nigeria, it was shown to be closely related to Rabies. The fruit bats I caught in numbers in mist nets in my garden were all examined in the laboratory but we never found a Vom Bat Virus. However with more specific reagents in later years, a host of strange viruses were isolated in West Africa after I left, from shrews and even insects; viruses with strange-sounding names like Mokola, Obodhiang and Kotonkan. Many were closely related to Rabies.

Such was the image conjured up by Rabies that veterinary officers when handling dogs usually took precautions which would have been considered unnecessary in countries where Rabies did not exist. Even the most docile dogs, whether vaccinated or not, were automatically muzzled with a tape before handling, particularly for any painful manipulation. Rubber gloves were worn for any examination of the mouth. Those who ignored these precautions, and there were one or two, paid the penalty with a painful course of injections.

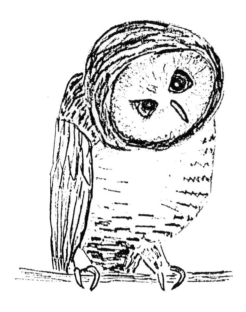

Young Marsh Owl

Lassie had me worried one Sunday evening when we returned from the weekly film shown at the Yelwa Club. Most unlike her not to greet us at the door, she was instead sitting up in the bedroom, salivating, lower jaw hanging open, looking decidedly miserable . . . in fact a clear cut case of dumb rabies was my first thought. She spent the night in the garage and looked a little better the next morning. I plucked up the courage to examine her mouth with gloves and found her tongue still swollen at the back. The problem was solved when Dantiyi produced a dead bee from the bedroom floor, with saliva still on it.

I learnt to be very careful handling virulent Rabies material in the laboratory. No preventative vaccinations were available in the early 1960s. Finding it impossible to wear gloves and satisfactorily hold a small syringe and an anaesthetised mouse, one tended to develop a careful technique with bare hands. With fingers and thumb only millimetres from the sharp point of the needle, those who were sloppy in their technique had to face up to a painful course of anti-rabies shots, because any accidental cut or needle-prick on the work bench had to be reported immediately.

Disposal of dog carcases infected with Rabies caused a problem or two. At first they were burnt in an old brick-built incinerator with a wide brick chimney, until a tragedy occurred. One of the locals, attracted by the smell of roasting dog meat, a great delicacy, climbed in through the chimney and was unable to get out before being overcome by smoke.

Later, carcases were soaked for twenty-four hours in bins containing a very crude Cresol or Phenol product, a particularly strong and evil-smelling disinfectant called Admiralty Fluid, before they were buried in a pit. One of the doctors at Vom Mission Hospital complained that he was treating patients for Phenol poisoning. Some dog carcases were being exhumed by members of his flock, so the pit was fenced and the gate kept under lock and key, yet even this was not an absolute deterrent.

Eventually an isolation block, containing an oil-fired carcase digester like an enormous pressure-cooker, surrounded by a high security fence with padlocked gates, at last provided safe disposal of infected carcases. In fact we could have opened a soup kitchen, had there been a demand, because the digested and well-sterilised broth ran to waste in a sump; little remained of the solids. This building also allowed us to work on other virulent diseases, like Rinderpest, without infected animals escaping.

In spite of her placid nature, our cat Pyewacket still liked to give the illusion of living dangerously. Occasionally she brought to the house small snakes, but never onto the bed, thank goodness. They wriggled around on the concrete floor till swept outside and most were quite harmless. The house snake, which squeezed its prey to death, was common around Vom and a bit of a nuisance in the laboratory mouse colony.

A delightful old Hausaman, Garba Daya, looked after the mouse colony and nothing pleased him more than to take children round on a Sunday morning. There were boxes and boxes of mice in tiers on racks. Sadly, white mice were required for other uses in the Laboratory besides Rabies. These small house snakes could wriggle into a mouse-box through the holes into which the water bottles were inserted, if any extra holes were left unblocked. The snakes dined handsomely on a mouse or two and then were prevented from getting out through the same hole by their bulging midriffs. I was pleased that Garba generally let them go outside.

Several species of venomous snakes like cobras, night adders, and a

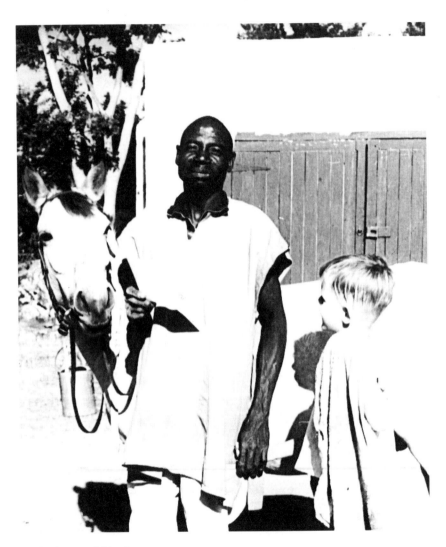

Garba Daya and friends

back-fanged tree snake, the boomslang, were about. Two variants were present in Vom, a dark brown and a green variety, and with one shot I demolished one of each entwined together obviously mating in a tree over our driveway. What a way to die -*in flagrante delicto*- but they were close to a sunbird's nest.

Other snakes, like a spitting cobra and a forest cobra, were shot when they came too near the house, as we were concerned for Roger's safety. The corpses were always welcomed by Gerry Dunger, a private medical practitioner in Jos, the same who climbed Wase Rock.

Gerry was an enthusiastic herpetologist who wrote several entertaining articles on snakes in the Journal of the Nigerian Field Society. His photographic illustrations were excellent. He handled lethal specimens with impunity, as we once witnessed on his lawn. While we remained in the safety of our car on his driveway, we watched him tweaking the tail of a spitting cobra to make it assume a suitable pose for photography; it was getting very angry indeed – spitting mad, in fact – I thought the term very appropriate.

We provided Gerry with his first specimen of the Forest Cobra from the Plateau. It had been in our roof dining on bats, for there were two bat carcases inside. It chose to descend to ground level down the front of our aviary just as June was attracted outside by the fluttering of its occupants, a pair of injured falcons.

June had an eye-to-eye confrontation with the cobra, which later measured nearly six feet, and was very lucky indeed not to get struck in the face. As I spread the corpse in the garage, Dantiyi got quite upset when I straightened the tail, insisting that snakes were dangerous at both ends. When I told him he had it wrong – only horses were dangerous at both ends and damned uncomfortable in the middle – he did not see the joke.

One evening at a Committee Meeting of the Nigerian Field Society in the Dunger residence in Jos, Gerry startled all of us present. Producing a small bag of snakes sent to him that day by a mission doctor up the Benue River, he took one out in his hand. They felt so small, he told us, that he was sure they were harmless. Then feeling the rough keeling on its scales, he realised it was a Saw-scaled Viper *Echis carinatus*, a small but very nasty customer which accounts for many deaths in north and tropical Africa and Asia, and dropped the lot on the floor. We all stood on chairs till he rounded them up.

There may have been many deaths due to snake-bite amongst Nigerians which we never heard about, but I recall Gerry telling me of only one case amongst expatriates and it was caused by this species. A child living near the Benue River was bitten on the foot and later died in the Jos Hospital.

Like many others I was loath to touch reptiles of any sort with bare hands, including the harmless geckoes and chameleons which were very common. Chameleons were thought by the locals to be venomous and Dantiyi would never touch one. The first I found was a most cooperative subject for photography, first in black and white, using a newly-acquired electronic flash, and later slow motion cine photography. It fed readily on beetles and moths placed in front of it, projecting its tongue about four inches, almost a third of its overall length.

Each year when the snipe arrived, Lassie and I explored wide expanses of grassland round Vom. Low-lying hollows became very swampy adjacent to where the snipe were. These swamps were treacherous places, with deep pools of water in which small minnow-sized fish could be caught with a fishing net made of gauze.

We discovered this before Roger came out for his first summer holidays, near the end of the wet season. Eager to keep Roger and his friends amused we dashed out to some of the more accessible swamps between heavy showers. We kept some very colourful fish in a 30 gallon aquarium which I bought from a friend who was leaving for good. They required no special aeration apparatus, only rain water and ant eggs. One group of fish, *Aphyosemion* species, were iridescent blue with red and gold markings and may have laid drought-resistent eggs, because during the dry season the swamps seemed to dry up.

During these fleeting excursions we sometimes flushed small attractive owls from the vicinity of these swamps They flew around inquisitively during the late afternoons, when their dark eye and chestnut panel on each wing could readily be seen. They were Marsh Owls, about which little was known, though Robert Gambles, Principal of the Vom Veterinary School, found a nest containing eggs in October, 1960, while hunting for dragonflies.

Later, at the start of the dry season, a friend of Dantiyi's offered me a young Marsh Owl, unable to fly, with primary feathers only half grown. He found it sitting in a dry clump of grass in one of these swamps and thought it had been abandoned. I kept it several months and it made a delightful pet, having the freedom of the house and flying around our

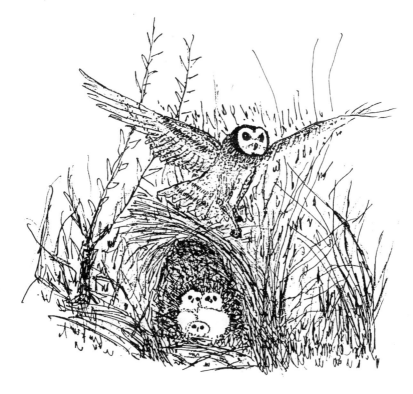

Marsh Owl leaving nest

large lounge during the evenings. It spent the rest of the time in an aviary I built for it along the side of the house under the eave.

Surplus white mice from the Laboratory colony were always available and these I killed and fed whole to the owl, an ideal natural food as owls in captivity must have roughage. They eject pellets of undigested fur and bones before feeding again. This young owl swallowed even adult mice whole, but met its match when it tried to do the same with the drumstick from a large cooked chicken, which I had only left nearby for it to play with. For twenty-four hours the poor bird looked decidedly uncomfortable, until I extracted the bone with forceps.

Realising this species of owl probably started to breed late in the wet season, I studied one of the nearby swamps, which was readily accessible from the roadside, looking for possible nest sites. Going out at dusk I took compass bearings on all the places where owls alighted. The following afternoon I would walk along these bearings, carefully watching where I put my feet. I found a number of nests by this method, mostly with eggs in them, and beside one nest Badung, our garden boy, helped me put up a hide of grass matting.

When the eggs hatched, a keen photographer, Bob Killick-Kendrick, took some excellent flash photographs, which appeared in an article we submitted to *Ibis*. Not to be outdone I took some cine film from the same hide, but this stretched my ingenuity a bit. A portable 240V generator at the roadside, 120 yards of cable, a rheostat and a 1000W photoflood bulb on the front of the hide, allowed me to sit in the hide with the rheostat on my knee, adjusted so the photoflood only glowed dull orange. Ignoring the alarming crackling noises it made, I could light up the whole swamp like daylight by turning the rheostat up, though goodness knows what any of the local natives thought of this almost supernatural spectacle. When the light was turned up slowly the owls accepted it and I was able to get some brief but very satisfying sequences on film.

Contrary to the scant facts known about this species, rats up to six inches long, caught nearby where crops were harvested, made up the diet and not insects as was supposed. The eggs hatched at two day intervals, and the adults enticed the older young from the nest to disperse them so as not to have all their eggs in one basket, so to speak. For a ground-nesting species, with nestlings unable to fend for themselves at hatching, this seemed a very sensible thing to do. Obviously the baby Marsh Owl given to me the previous year had not been abandoned.

The aviary built along the side of the house for the first baby Marsh Owl, which died of an accident after five months, became a sort of convalescent home for injured birds of prey. The moonflower creeper growing up the wire netting provided dense cover, turning the aviary into a very secluded retreat. Word got around that I was interested in owls, and I must confess I had a very soft spot for them.

An adult White-faced Scops Owl, the most beautiful of all the smaller owls, with orange eyes in a white facial disc bordered with black, and a grey-brown vermiculated plumage, became the first patient. An abscess on the shoulder prevented it from flying. I suspected a catapult injury, because native children were good shots and often destructively smashed the mud nests of swallows and rock-martins under bridges, for instance. A week later the abscess burst, allowing the owl to make short flights, so I let it go. For a night or two it returned for the dead mouse I left out for it.

Owls were considered good *Ju-Ju* by Africans and live ones were often offered for sale in the markets. An African Barn Owl, which a friend bought in Jos market, became my longest patient. Every primary wing feather had been pulled out and they never grew again, for I believe the follicles were damaged beyond repair. He ate regularly and found himself a secluded corner which he jealously guarded. He eyed all other temporary patients with great distrust, swaying rhythmically when he felt at all threatened. He looked rather ludicrous with his flightless wings and the other patients gave him a wide berth, no doubt thinking he had some horrible disease.

An adult Spotted Eagle-Owl, unable to fly with an injured wing, also came my way. This large but gentle owl allowed me to examine its wing, which was not broken though badly bruised at the elbow – undoubtedly a catapult again. With no treatment except rest and several mice, it made a rapid recovery. A few days after admission Pyewacket walked past trailing her coat. The eagle owl, on the ground at the time, put on an impressive threat display, fanning and arching both wings and lowering its head so that it looked like a huge boulder. Obviously the injured wing had healed, so I left the aviary door open. For several weeks it hung around the garden spending the day in our mango tree.

By contrast the smallest, a European Scops Owl, almost fitted into the palm of my hand. It was one of several migrant owls which I caught by mist-net and ringed and kept in the aviary just for the day.

I also was given several young owls of different species. I reared two young Marsh Owls from a large litter of six and took them to Edinburgh Zoo, where they survived for several years. They travelled with us when

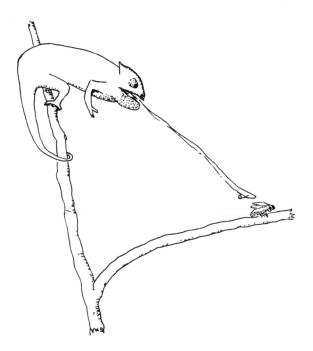

Chameleon feeding

we went on leave. I had made arrangements to fly Jos-Kano-London-Glasgow so we could collect a car for our leave. By a fortuitous stroke of luck Heathrow airport was fog-bound and the Boeing 707 from Kano was diverted to Prestwick near Glasgow, where we got off, though not without difficulty as the BOAC staff had to find our luggage. Collecting the car, we drove to Edinburgh, dropped off the two owls and then down to Moffat, arriving there much earlier than expected.

Other injured birds of prey found my aviary a convalescent haven. A Red-tailed Buzzard, a Lanner falcon and a Shikra were all returned to the wild when they recovered, though I kept the Lanner several weeks during my last tour trying to train it for falconry. Hit by a taxi on the road, it had been stunned. Two of the outer primary wing feathers on one side were broken but grew again. Unfortunately my time ran out with approaching final departure so I 'hacked him back to the wild' as the old falconry expression goes.

Lanner falcons were not considered bold enough for serious falconry, yet once, while enjoying a walk with Hil Fry and Dave Ebbutt, we witnessed an impressive display of their capabilities, which Dave wrote up as a short communication in the *Nigerian Ornithologist's Bulletin*. A pair of Lanner falcons regularly nested on Kafo Rock, guarding their territory jealously. We were watching from a distance, when the smaller male stooped at a Pied Crow, which was flying past quite innocently several hundred yards from the nest site. It seemed to be a mock attack, yet the Pied Crow tumbled out of the sky and was dead when we picked it up a few minutes later. When we examined the dead crow, its liver had ruptured and the abdomen was full of blood, sufficient explanation for its rapid death. However a small bruise on the back of the skull indicated it had been stunned first by a blow to the head, and the liver rupture and haemorrhage were probably a result of the ground impact.

CHAPTER 6

Game Parks and Local Customs

IN MAY 1963 ROGER WAS TO START AT MY OLD BOARDING SCHOOL Greenways at the beginning of the summer term and I planned my leave that year so that June and I could be near at hand during his first term. When we booked Roger I was surprised to learn that the dear old soul, who had been wife of the headmaster in my day, still ran the school. She offered us a cottage on the school grounds for part of my leave and we spent a delightful few weeks near Warminster in Wiltshire, not far from Salisbury Plain and Stonehenge.

We solved the problem of transport whilst on this leave in an ingenious way. A colleague in Vom, Ian Macadam, offered me at a very reasonable price an old Rover 60, which he had used during his last leave. I had to collect it in Glasgow, which suited me fine as it was on the occasion I delivered two owls to Edinburgh Zoo. Before departing on leave I had already arranged to pass on the same car to another couple going on leave from Jos when we finished with it. They had the same trouble-free motoring we had for four months.

Soon after the Christmas festivities in 1962, as a treat for Roger before he started boarding school, we took ourselves to a game park before we all went on leave. The nearest well-established park, Waza Game Reserve, was about 700 miles away in the French Cameroons south of Lake Chad. We were told it was well worth a visit, so in January I was granted a few days off, ostensibly to look at the disease threat posed by wild animals, and we joined two other families, the Godfreys and the Kil-lick-Kendricks also heading that way. Altogether there were six adults and six children in our party and with spare room in our car we decided to take Dantiyi. Although we were away from Vom for a week, four

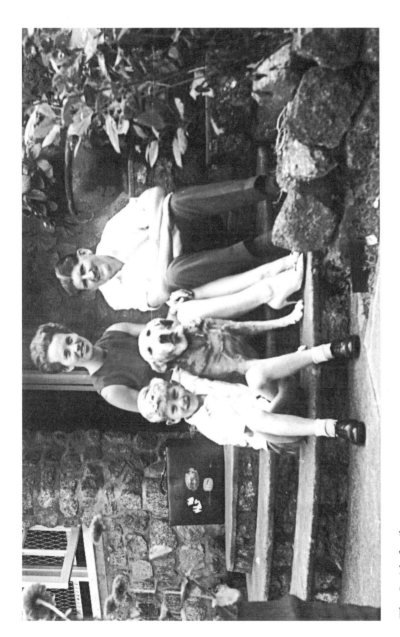

The Smith family

days were spent travelling to and fro, partly over the same road I had travelled at the end of my first tour.

We left Vom early in the morning with Dantiyi's rather large bedding roll on the roofrack, the only place we could put it. Alas, I realised before we had got too far down the track that we would never make the trip at 40 m.p.h. all the way, the best speed my little Fiat 110 could achieve with such an encumbrance. The wind resistance influenced our car's performance severely, so back to Vom we went, where we unloaded not only the bedding roll but regretfully Dantiyi also, deciding that we could not separate the two. We would have to fend for ourselves as best we could. We still reached Potiskum, about half way to our night stop, in time for lunch with the others.

Our first night in Maiduguri was a shambles as our bookings had gone astray. Such a mix-up was not an infrequent event in Nigeria. After travelling 400 miles we were not at all amused to find that the Catering Rest House was absolutely full and we had to split up – I eventually found a bed with the Provincial Veterinary Officer, Forrest Laing, after he had helped me find beds for everyone else.

The next morning we found the road to Bama was a superb highway, obviously built as an inducement to the inhabitants of that region to side with Nigeria rather than join the French Cameroons. That bit of disputed territory lay on the border.

Arriving at Waza late on the afternoon of our second day out of Vom, we shared delightful little four-bed rondavels on a prominent hill outside the Game Reserve and made daily visits to the reserve by car. A long serviceable dry-weather airstrip near the base camp obviously catered for visitors from further afield.

The tracks through the bush were prepared by grader but were not rolled, thus they were not kind to the tyres on our cars. In low lying places the stumps of the coarse elephant grass were sharp and strong enough to spike the tyres, even steel-reinforced Michelin X. Although we only had one puncture, our companions spent a lot of time changing wheels and repairing tyres. The tracks linked water holes and at two of them hides were erected in trees. On our last morning before dawn I took the ladies to one of them hoping to see elephant as there were abundant tracks in the mud, but we were out of luck.

This was our first visit to a game reserve. Two unusual animal species in this rather out-of-the-way place were Reticulated Giraffe and Topi or Korigum, one of the hartebeests. Of both we saw many at close quarters and they all looked remarkably healthy, posing no threat to domestic livestock, which were not allowed into the reserve anyway.

The orchard bush was fairly open, with little undergrowth in places, and at first we tended to train our eyes at ground level, looking for signs of life beneath the canopy, until we rather unexpectedly saw the head of a giraffe nearby peering down at us over the top of an acacia. It allowed very close approach, yet its dappled legs were remarkably difficult to see, even when we knew where to look. We saw only one elephant which we stalked in the bush, feeling very brave, though all the poor beast wanted to do was get away from us. Several warthog had families of tiny piglets which played follow-my-leader, all with their tails stiffly erect like little flagpoles, each with a tuft of hair on top.

Most of the time June drove slowly along the tracks through the bush, with Roger in the front passenger seat, while I sat in the back eagerly filming out of both back windows. We passed a few bushbuck, but saw none of the large carnivores, though we knew there were lion in the reserve. At one waterhole where we all piled out of our cars to have a picnic, I had that uneasy feeling that we were being watched.

Of birds we saw many, including ostriches, hundreds of crowned cranes, large bustards and several unusual Secretary Birds stalking sedately through the bush. We eagerly approached several White-backed Vultures in a tall tree near one of the waterholes, but they had picked the kill bare and all that remained were a few large bones. Bateleur Eagles were common, easy to identify in flight because their feet protrude behind their short tails.

Our three nights in the camp and reserve passed all too quickly, but on our way back through the border into Nigeria, we collected several bottles of *Vin Ordinaire*, presumably French Algerian wine, which we found very palatable at the price.

The first Nigerian Game Park was only opened in 1962 at Yankari beyond Bauchi and south of the Gombe road. Over 700 square miles in area, it straddled the Gaji River. A former Veterinary Officer with the Northern Region Veterinary Services, Robert Coulthard, was appointed the first Regional Game Warden in 1955, but he died in 1961 and was succeeded by Mallam Jibrin Jia.

We were not given the chance to visit Yankari Game Park until a year before we left Nigeria when June and I accompanied a team from the Institute for Trypanosomiasis Research in Vom, who spent a few days at Yankari trying to dart animals using a crossbow. They intended to collect blood samples from the anaesthetised beasts so that they could study trypanosomiasis in wild game animals, but their weapon was hopelessly inaccurate. Young village boys, I am sure, could have taught them a thing or two about accuracy with their catapults. I had hoped to scrounge a drop or two of blood from any wild animals they sampled, so that I could carry out assays on viral antibodies, but I cannot recall any being sampled.

The bush in Yankari was too thick for comfortable viewing even though we sat on benches in the back of their Forward Control Land Rover and had the benefit of an elevated viewing platform. However at a distance we saw dwarf West African Buffalo, known as Bush-cow, the most feared game animal in West Africa, and frightened several antelope with the crossbow. Tsetse flies were abundant, as this bit of riverine territory favoured them, and I made what I was sure was an interesting observation. The flies seemed to prefer African skins to our white ones and if *Bature* sat still we were hardly bothered. Nothing new in that, I was told by the pundits. When they are feeding, the tsetse flies prefer the darker shaded areas on the under side of animals.

The big attraction at Yankari Game Park was the Wikki Warm Spring after which the base camp was named. Beneath the campsite, thousands of gallons an hour of warm water surged from a large cave at the bottom of a sandstone cliff and ran down a watercourse over gravel to join the Gaji River. The water was very refreshing indeed, but by the time we staggered up the two hundred steps back to the base camp, we were invariably in a lather again.

The warm spring at Wikki indicated thermal activity not far below the ground and was one of several interesting geological features to be found in central Nigeria. The huge trachyte plug called Wase Rock was to the south of Yankari. On the Plateau, within comfortable range of Vom for day trips, a number of other geological features allowed me to brush up on my amateur geology.

The ancient granites of the Plateau, which by weathering made up the fluvio-volcanic plains in which the alluvial miners found tin and associated minerals, were intruded by much more recent volcanic activity. Vom itself was built in and around a weathered volcanic cinder cone,

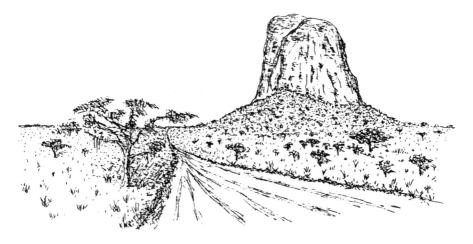

Wase Rock

but visible to the west at Miango was a more perfect cinder cone, hardly weathered at all. At the south end of the Plateau a cluster of similar cones were readily visible and the southernmost one contained a crater lake, supposedly occupied by sacred crocodiles.

The road south to Pankshin passed through the impressive Mongu Dyke, an intrusion of volcanic magma which stood out like a gigantic palisade on either side of the road. On the western side of the Plateau near Ropp at a place called Dutsan Umat, a volcanic plug intruded less impressively than Wase Rock, but its fine-grained trachyte rock contained similar crystals of sanadine and inclusions of older granite and there were caves on one side.

During our last couple of years in Vom, a Polish geologist, Carol Paulo, showed us many of these features and, by giving me small samples, he interested me in some of the minerals found on the Plateau. He worked for ATMN and once showed me round the assay laboratory in Bukuru where my perverted sense of humour made me wonder whether some of their equipment, with names like primary and secondary jigs, shaking tables, mechanical screens and airfloats could not have been more appropriately utilised in a bordello.

They were all necessary to separate the alluvial minerals which were found in association with tin to a varying degree. The tin concentrate, separated from most of the lighter worthless material by its specific gravity, contained only about 70% cassiterite, the main tin ore, which occurred in a number of different forms and colours. Early prospectors found quite large nuggets and Roger Harrison gave me one, surprisingly heavy for its size, which made a fine paperweight, though most of the tin mined commercially was in the form of a fine powder. Small quantities of columbite, zircon, monazite (which contained radio-active thorium), fergusonite and xenotine were also present. In some deposits gem quality topaz, tourmaline, beryl, garnets and zircons could be found. These were more common where the tin lay in pegmatites, intrusive bodies containing large crystals which seemed to enrich the quality of the minerals present.

Near Jos at one tin mine, a huge hole in the ground beside which the overburden lay in untidy mountains, water jets were used to wash out the tin-bearing soil, a process known as hydraulicking. Gravel pumps sucked up the sludge into settling tanks. Only tin ore, columbite and the rarer minerals were retained in the concentrate. Discarded in huge waste dumps were piles of semi-precious quartz and topaz, also heaps of black ilmenite and rutile, a source of titanium. The topaz was water-worn, usually badly flawed and worthless.

The open-cut tin mines were a dreadful eyesore, but the Mines Reclamation Unit did try with its limited resources to restore areas which were worked out, by planting the huge piles of overburden with a legume, which returned some nitrogen to the impoverished earth and allowed further planting of trees.

Flows of basalt lava over the deeper alluvial tin deposits interfered with their mining and required specialised techniques. On the leases of a small mining company at Makafo, where lived our friends John and Barbara Clark, the Arim River had cut across and exposed a basalt lava flow which ages ago had cooled sufficiently slowly to form the perfect hexagonal columns of a miniature Giant's Causeway.

It was at Makafo, while visiting the Clarks, that we once witnessed the extraordinary sight of migrating Fulani on the move, heading south at the beginning of the dry season. Several families were spaced out along the line of march, which stretched almost out of sight in each direction. Each family with its animals moved along the route at a steady pace, the bulls carrying their worldly possessions. Young animals were sometimes carried by the menfolk and the women and children all had pots or bedding to carry. It seemed to be a remarkably well-organised exercise. At their destination, they would quickly weave *Zana* mats and make their traditional grass hut, *Rumfa*, with materials which lay at hand.

During the wet season on the Plateau the Fulani sold their milk to the Plateau Dairy which provided collection points in the larger villages and a lorry which did the rounds. The Plateau Dairy, not far from the Laboratories in Vom, prepared butter and cheese. Nothing was wasted.

The skim milk was dried and the powder fortified with ground-nut meal and sold as a baby food called Arlac. Our biochemist in Vom, Frank Peers, examined the batches of ground-nut meal for evidence of a fungal contaminant, aflotoxin. This was the toxin produced by a species of *Aspergillus flavus*, a fungus which grew on cereal foodstuffs under conditions of high humidity and temperature. It readily grew on ground-nuts when they were stored improperly and allowed to get damp, and at the railhead at Kano where thousands of bags of ground-nuts were stored in huge pyramids, it was always a race against time to get them railed south for shipment overseas before the onset of the wet season. The high incidence of liver cancer in West Africans was attributed to this highly carcinogenic toxin. Frank once showed me some wizened nuts, which apparently the ground-nut sorters considered a great delicacy. They were so rich in aflotoxin that they fluoresced under his Ultraviolet Lamp.

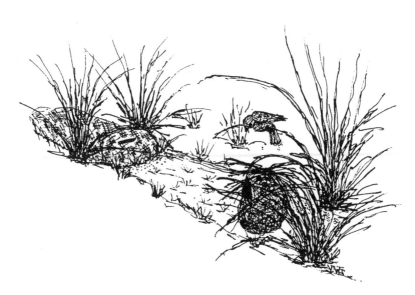

Orange Bishop's nest and hide

An important viral disease of cattle about which we did little until near the end of my stay in Nigeria, was Foot and Mouth Disease (FMD). We knew several strains or types of the virus existed in Nigeria – at least four – and I had already seen the consequences of a small outbreak in Lagos. In developed countries FMD was greatly feared, because it caused tremendous economic loss and its significance could therefore be measured in such terms.

The fever and blistering in the mouth and on the feet make milking cows go off their milk. Beef animals lose weight and young calves or piglets may die. The virus is tough and, unlike the Rinderpest virus, can survive for long periods in animal products. However FMD is not a major killer like Rinderpest, though its causative virus, related to that which causes the common cold, is one of the most infectious agents known in animals.

The disease seemed to smoulder amongst the Fulani cattle. When detected by field veterinary staff samples were collected and sent to us for onward transmission to the Reference Laboratory at Pirbright in Britain for typing, so that the distribution of the four known types could be plotted and constantly monitored.

All the cattle in the infected herd were then deliberately infected by swabbing their mouths with infectious material, a procedure known as mouthing. This minimised the period of quarantine and ensured that all the animals developed antibodies. Of obvious disease there were often no signs at all in some of the animals.

The only animals under serious threat were those of improved breeds in government farms. Although well segregated from native Fulani herds, we were always worried that FMD disease might break out in these valuable animals, if adequate precautions were not maintained. Vaccination was the answer, but before this could be done trials were necessary to test the efficacy of various FMD vaccines.

When the former Director, Ian Taylor, left Vom, he joined the Wellcome Foundation in Britain, one of the major producers of FMD vaccine. He suggested a small trial should be carried out in cattle at our Livestock Investigation Centre, using vaccines prepared from the various types of FMD virus known to occur in Nigeria. After Ian vaccinated the several groups of cattle, he returned to Britain and I attended to the subsequent serial blood sampling of the animals to test how long their antibodies lasted. Amongst the groups of cattle were some which received combined FMD vaccine and rinderpest vaccine simultaneously. Always mindful of the need to minimise handling of animals in the field, the combination of several different vaccines administered at the same time was frequently assessed, but it was always necessary to ensure that one vaccine did not interfere with the other. Rinderpest vaccine had been previously tried with Bovine Pleuro-pneumonia vaccine.

The FMD vaccine trial was considered successful, but I remember one cow which received all four types in one shot, did develop rather alarming vesicles or blisters in her mouth, which soon healed. The obvious solution was not to use four types simultaneously.

Our farm LIC was well equipped with a cattle race and crush so that if we were using farm animals for any trials they could be run through and blood samples taken with minimum fuss. At the farm I had calves under test also, so quite frequently visited the place to collect samples. Identification of individual animals depended on a complicated series of notches on their ears, which I found hard to interpret.

Reading the numbers was no problem for one of the LIC staff, a small Ibo, for that reason nicknamed Samson, who was always present when we had to identify animals. Cheerful, bright as a button, he had been born and bred in Vom. I was very saddened to learn only a few months after I left Vom, that he was one of the many hundreds of Ibos massacred on the Plateau. Apparently he refused to leave his post.

Until the Massacre of the Ibos happened in late 1966, many expatriates would have found it hard to believe that such dreadful internecine strife could possibly happen in a country which looked so stable, a country which was often quoted as an example of African democracy. Yet even while we lived there during those few happy post-independence years, we did not have to look far below the surface to recognise that there simmered an unhappy state of affairs, that ethnic minorities felt threatened, that dominant parties seemed to rule the roost. By 1964 Nigeria had become a Republic within the Commonwealth, yet the Nigerian people showed enormous diversity, not only in the many different tribal groups which had made up the four regions of the former Federation, but also in their customs, religions and attitudes to life.

Expatriates who were eager to learn of the many different life-styles of the natives were encouraged to become members of the Nigerian Field Society, which had been founded by A. F. B. Bridges in 1930, an organisation devoted to the study of West Africa, its plants, animals and environment, its people and their culture The monthly meetings of the Jos branch, and several Provincial Centres had branches, were well attended and there were regular outings to the field throughout the year.

Members also received quarterly a well-illustrated printed journal which contained articles on the history and customs of some of the local tribes, mingled with others on the flora and fauna, several on birds and such diverse subjects as hawkmoths, reptiles, dragonflies or fish. Some articles on geology and mining, climate, neighbouring countries, early exploration or even reminiscences of the past, the 'good old days' for those who survived, made the journal quite fascinating to read and a useful vehicle in which many an eccentric expatriate, like myself, propounded his interests or views, in my case on birds breeding around Vom.

However, one did not have to read the *Nigerian Field* or attend their meetings to be aware of strange customs all around. Even on the Plateau those of the local tribal groups showed great diversity. An event which was usually well-attended by spectators was a Fulani Beating, at which the Fulani youngsters showed their endurance to pain. It was their initiation into manhood, and they invited adult members of their family and others to beat them with wooden staves, but there were rules. Seemingly the blows could not be struck below the waist or above the shoulders, but any flinch or cry was greeted with derision. It was no fanciful staged affair. The blows were laid on with a lot of force.

Another form of entertainment could be witnessed in the extreme south of the Plateau on the escarpment, where a very primitive pagan tribe lived at a village called Richa. The men-folk differed in their ceremonial dress, in that instead of the grass penis-shields worn by some pagan men elsewhere, the Richa pagans used cow horns secured erect by leather thongs.

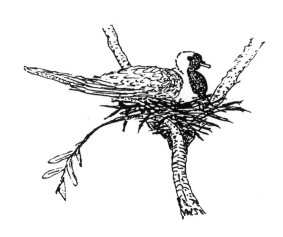

Male Long-Tailed Dove on nest

It seemed to delight some female visitors to have their photographs taken alongside such handsomely-dressed fellows. The pagans would perform a dance if sufficient visitors arrived, so it was worthwhile to make up a group to justify the trip. If the visit coincided with one of their frequent binges on the home-brewed atcha beer, it was a spectacle well worth attending.

By contrast the Hausa were dignified and deeply religious Mohammedans, praying five times a day. It was part of their contract that they be allowed to do so, and during work breaks they would discreetly withdraw with their prayer mats for a few minutes devotions, facing east to Mecca. During the month-long fast of Ramadan, no food or water could be taken during daylight hours so before dawn they would take a full meal to last them the day. Little wonder that their energy seemed to fade by mid-afternoon. A number of the Hausa staff, who had served in the forces during the war, were a little bit more emancipated.

There were, of course, Moslem festivals throughout the year, such as at the end of Ramadan or on the Prophet's birthday, when sheep or goats were slaughtered by having their throats cut in front of their house.

These festivals were celebrated by all and sundry along with the other Christian festivals, so that the laboratory staff did fairly well for holidays, not that we were always able to take them, because of work constraints. Using animals for trials or vaccine production was one thing, as their care and feeding could always be attended to by junior staff. On the other hand tissue cultures, cultures of living cells in bottles, also required feeding but needed much more careful handling to avoid bacteriological contamination or stress. I zealously and selfishly preferred to look after my own, even if it meant foregoing a holiday.

My fame as an ardent photographer of birds at their nests spread and a call from Dr. Zwilling, the Manager of the Fish Farm at Panyam, sent me down there hotfoot one weekend. He had found a Green-backed Heron's nest with three nestlings in a sparse platform of twigs built in a willow tree growing over the water of one of the tanks and had very kindly set up for me a grass-matting hide overlooking the nest. The proximity of the water encouraged hordes of mosquitoes which ate me alive the following weekend as I tried unsuccessfully to sleep in my little Fiat, but at least I was in the hide before daybreak, and spent several hours watching the parent birds feed the youngsters with quite large fish, while they clambered precariously around the branches. The staff of the Fish Farm did not seem to begrudge the birds helping themselves to a few fish.

The Fish Farm began as an experiment in the mid-1950s to provide fish as a source of protein for the locals. That included us in Vom, where we were regularly offered the choice of Niger Perch – *Giwan Ruwa* – quite delicious, relatively bone-free but very expensive because it grew slowly, or bony European Carp, a bit like cotton wool and as tasteless, or delicious *Tilapia* species. Unfortunately the more popular edible fish did not breed very successfully, so the poorer quality fish usually won the day.

The large artificially-created ponds were set attractively amongst tall

Borassus (Fan) palms in which piapiacs or black magpies nested. In the top of a very high dead trunk, from which the crown had detached, I remember a pair of grey kestrels had their nest. During the dry season the Fish Farm was a pleasant place for a picnic. Tables and benches were provided beneath thatched cover. The green vegetation around the open ponds provided a perfect contrast to the parched, dry and rocky countryside elsewhere on the Plateau.

One had to be careful around many of the open expanses of water on the Plateau, like the mining dams. If effluent from nearby native villages drained into the water, the risk of contracting schistosomiasis (bilharziasis) was great, particularly if the snails which acted as intermediate hosts for this parasitic blood-fluke were also present. The larvae penetrated through human skin, so it was inadvisable to paddle or swim in water known to be infected, as the course of treatment was unpleasant. There was a high incidence of this disease amongst the native population of the Plateau.

The guinea-worm, an even more horrendous parasite with the ghastly name *Dracunculus medinensis*, was more prevalent along the major rivers but not unknown on the Plateau. Its life cycle was dependant on a small water flea which had to be swallowed. Other parasites were common near running water and one place we were always warned about was Assob Falls, a local beauty spot at the foot of the escarpment on the road to Lagos. Onchocerciasis or River-blindness was caused by a little filarial parasite which got in the eye and was spread by a small biting fly, very commonly found around Assob.

At college I had avidly read all about these dreadful parasites and even memorised their long names, never expecting to meet them face-to-face, so to speak. I found it quite astonishing when I finally left Nigeria, that with all my activities chasing after birds in and near water I was very fortunate never to have contracted any of these nasty diseases. Or perhaps it was not a matter of good luck but good care, although on one memorable occasion I neglected to protect myself while wading in the pool near Kafo filming the birdlife and was savagely attacked by leeches. Most of them I removed, but blood was still flowing freely down my legs when I returned home in time to interrupt one of June's afternoon tea-parties.

Care with health and hygiene, of course, did not stop out in the bush. Around many of the mining dams where there was plentiful water, native gardeners grew fine crops of vegetables for sale to the Europeans. In the village markets and even in Jos near the large Kingsway supermarket, many salad vegetables, like tomatoes, cucumbers, radishes and lettuce, were displayed in beautiful array by traders. What the trader never told you was that the vegetables were grown in plots fertilised with 'Night soil' from the native quarters, in other words human excrement. Hookworm infections and amoebic dysentery were also quite prevalent amongst the natives, so I found the thought and association quite distasteful.

If one still wished to eat vegetables normally eaten uncooked, they had to be carefully washed in clean water, that is boiled and filtered

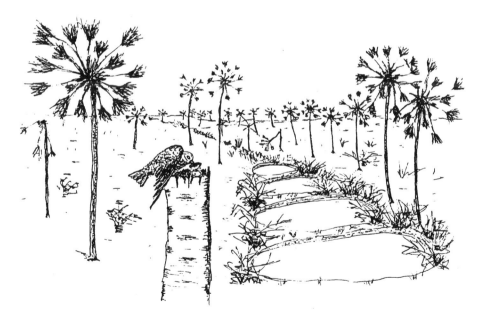

Grey Kestrel's nest at Panyam

water, or soaked in disinfectant, usually a hypochlorite like Milton, or the ubiquitous 'Pot Permang.'

As a virologist I was aware of all these hazards to healthy living as a matter of course, but there is one area in which I still consider myself extremely fortunate. Africa and South America have always been considered wonderful places in which new Arthropod-borne viruses were turning up constantly when anyone took the trouble to look. But many other very unpleasant viruses have emerged from Africa in the past thirty years, real killer viruses, like Marburg, Ebola, Lassa Fever (the first case in an expatriate occurred in Jos just after we left), the rabies-related Mokola, and more recently the HIV causing AIDS.

CHAPTER 7

Laboratory Staff and Visitors

IN VOM WE LIVED IN WHAT WAS PROBABLY THE HEALTHIEST PART OF NIGERIA, yet eighteen months tours still seemed a long time to go without a decent break. When I first went out, mid-tour local leaves were permitted and often taken by those who worked in less healthy parts of the country, but not long after Independence these were abolished. Government Hill Station on the outskirts of Jos, our nearby Provincial Centre, had been established for just such leaves, but living as we did on the Plateau only sixteen miles from Jos, the abolition of local leave had little effect on us. Yet towards the end of each tour of eighteen months many of the expatriate laboratory staff were inclined towards the usual 'end-of-tour' feeling that beset many Europeans working in Nigeria. On the other hand teaching staff, such as the Veterinary Education Officers at Vom Veterinary School, worked a three-term school year and were fortunate to be able to take shorter leaves after a tour of only nine or ten months.

Outward manifestations of this 'end-of-tour' feeling were few, but I generally felt stale and became quick-tempered with junior staff, often over some trivial matter. When the time came around to prepare the inevitable 'Handing-over notes,' so much a part of pre-leave preparations, my mood always lifted a bit. These notes were necessary to ensure the smooth functioning of a laboratory during temporary absences on leave. In the notes, after commenting on staff and projects in progress and listing reagents or vaccine stocks in hand or in preparation, some officers prescribed exactly what they wanted done, or not done, not that the incoming officer always paid much attention to such individual whims. The notes, duly signed by both parties, were to my way of thinking a sort of guaranteed insurance that if something dreadful happened during my absence, at least I could wave the notes in front of someone and say, 'Well, that's how it was before I left.'

The long leaves after relatively short tours, one of the apparent delights of service in West Africa, (after all, my father had endured four year tours pre-war in India), had one distinct disadvantage. No matter how diligently one saved up money during each tour, the funds rarely lasted the whole leave. Rarely could I afford to take my whole leave entitlement, so usually asked to return early, thus saving part as deferred leave. On two occasions I took the alternative option by doing short study courses during leave, as there was always ample need for brushing up on newer techniques.

In place of the first-class air fares to which we were entitled, we could instead apply for what was called an abnormal route allowance, which was in fact the cash equivalent of the first-class fare. By flying at a cheaper rate, one could make much longer journeys with a stopover in one or two interesting places.

For instance, at the end of my second tour, I took this allowance and we spent a month trying our hand at winter-sports in Switzerland and the Black Forest in southern Germany. What a contrast we noticed between the temperature of 112°F on the tarmac at Kano airport when we departed and the foot of snow we stepped into only a few hours later at Zurich airport. I had some justification for my visit there as I had been asked to have a chat with a Swiss girl from Zurich who had applied for a Technologist's position in Vom. Unfortunately her qualifications were not recognised by the Nigerian Government, a shame because she was an intelligent and capable girl who went out of her way, after I had interviewed her in the hotel, to take us to a huge department store where she helped us fully kit ourselves for the rigours of an Alpine winter.

During my last leave before we finally departed from Nigeria, I again took advantage of the abnormal route allowance. June and I visited Egypt and Greece. Roger by this time was at boarding school in England. The Chifneys, formerly from Vom, with whom we had enjoyed such chatty bridge evenings before their departure, were now in Cairo, Stan on an

F. A. O. appointment. They were one of several families from Vom with whom we have kept in touch. Nowadays I find it hard to explain the lasting friendships we made with families in Vom, yet some have endured for over thirty years. Perhaps it was because we were all much the same age, with young families and with much the same interests.

In Cairo, during those few days in late 1964, we were feted by the Chifneys and did all the things which tourists normally do in Egypt, but assisted greatly by having our own personal guide. I also took some ticks which I had recovered from migrant birds in Vom to a world authority on ticks, Harry Hoogstraal, who was at that time running an American Medical Research Unit (NAMRU–3) in Cairo. He kindly identified them for me. All were first stage nymphs of *Hyalomma marginata* and it seemed that they had probably been picked up by the birds after they had arrived south of the desert. I recall thinking at the time that if birds were parasitised by ticks, some of which carried blood-borne diseases, perhaps I should in future examine birds I netted to see if they were carrying parasites in their blood.

In March 1965 I returned for my last tour, which proved to be an eventful one. Having remained in Nigeria for five years after Independence, I felt I had trained Nigerian professional and technical staff as well as I could to take over the Virology Division, of which I was now the officer-in-charge. However I noticed with a sense of foreboding that some of my Nigerian colleagues, all of whom had obtained their veterinary qualifications overseas, seemed to be unwilling to accept responsibility.

In my Division there were also six Technologists, all bar one being Nigerian, the exception being Les Rowe, who had been seconded on contract for one tour to attend to matters pertaining to the rinderpest eradication scheme (JP 15). The remaining Nigerians had all started their training in Vom, but had completed their five year course of the Institute of Medical Laboratory Technology in Britain, returning fully trained, as

A.I.M.L.T.s. The first to return, even before I went to Vom, had been Jide Shonekan, who helped Reg Early train subsequent Technologists during their first two years. He took over the training programme from Reg when he retired.

In Vivien Oreffo, who married an Irish girl, Phil, while training as a Technologist in England, I had a strong right-hand man amongst the Nigerians. He helped me with tissue cultures and was a capable worker and an exceedingly pleasant fellow to work with. Only once did I have a slight altercation with him. One evening he took home keys to one of our coldrooms in which I had some cases of beer cooling for an evening function at Vom Club. If it happened again I threatened to lock him in the coldroom overnight, but later regretted my impulsive outburst for it almost reduced him to tears.

The several coldrooms we had around the laboratory were designed mainly for the storage of cartons of vaccines and other perishables. These were stacked on shelves and racks against the walls, leaving little floor space, though a few cases of beer could always be fitted in somewhere. The narrow doors to each coldroom limited access, yet on rare occasions one found the strangest objects inside.

In the coldroom nearest my office and adjacent to the front door of the Virology Laboratory, I stored many of the more valuable batches of seed vaccines, important reagents and vaccines which had already been tested and passed for issue. One Monday morning near the end of my second last tour, the 'end-of-tour' feeling strong upon me, I entered this coldroom and stumbled over a dead horse on the floor, its legs vertically upwards in the narrow passage way and cartons of precious vaccines balanced precariously on the hooves.; So rigid was the carcase set in *rigor mortis* it had to be dismembered to get it out again. What a gory mess had resulted. It was one of the school horses which had died on the Sunday morning, of a twisted bowel if I remember correctly.

One of my Senior Technologists, an Ibo named Cookey, with whom I never had cordial relations even at the best of times, but who usually did a satisfactory job looking after Rabies matters, had been Duty Technologist over that weekend and was responsible for what I took to be a personal vendetta against me, though in hindsight he had acted in good faith but had just chosen the wrong coldroom.

It was probably the only occasion on which I disregarded cordial Anglo-Nigerian relations. We were not supposed to speak crossly to our staff, yet I took my fury out on him, and we stood face to face while a group of interested Nigerian bystanders gathered around. I think most of them sided with me, for Cookey was not popular amongst the Hausa staff. He was downright argumentative most of the time, but on this occasion Cookey's little goatee beard, which I was often tempted to pull, fairly quivered as I explained the folly of his ways. I must have exercised considerable self-restraint, for if we had come to blows I would probably have been on the next plane home. AFRICA ALWAYS WINS.

Later, Cookey was selected for a short course in the United States to study immunofluorescent techniques for the diagnosis of Rabies. He went to the Communicable Diseases Centre in Atlanta, Georgia and I hoped the experience would improve his outlook on life, but he came back more obnoxious than ever.

Jonah, another Senior Laboratory Technologist, who looked after poultry vaccines and the rather mundane routine production of Lapinised and Caprinised Rinderpest Vaccines, was stolid and dependable, though he sometimes showed little initiative when things went wrong. As things went wrong with monotonous regularity, and equipment regularly broke down in spite of the capable administrations of Jack Dale, O. B. E., our Maintenance Superintendent, I always looked upon Jonah's appearance in the doorway of my office with foreboding. When he came to tell me an egg incubator had broken down and a batch of vaccine destroyed or some other disaster, I must have regarded him in the same suspicious way his namesake had been viewed by his shipmates.

I often wondered how Geoffrey Ibeachum, another Technologist, got his name and whether it had been a cruel joke by some 'Old Coaster' who had given his family the name, I-be-a-chum. He helped with the poultry vaccines and supervised the preparation of the considerable amount of equipment and glassware we constantly required.

Orage, a happy individual, who always seemed to be smiling, joined me only a short time before I left, but I remember him mainly because he bought my little Fiat 1100. Friends who remained after we departed often commented on how our old car appeared to have forgotten the rules of the road.

In spite of good technical staff, constant supervision of the junior staff was necessary in the laboratory, where several unwritten rules had to be observed. One of these was the destruction by breaking of all empty vials of antibiotics, otherwise they finished up in Vom village where they were filled with dirty water and sold by the local witch-doctor as a sure-fire cure for venereal disease, a remarkably common complaint amongst the locals (The Hausa words for the common cold and gonorrhoea are the same), with the undesirable emergence of antibiotic-resistant strains. We used a fair amount of penicillin and streptomycin in vaccines to minimise bacterial contamination and also in most tissue culture reagents.

Some of the junior staff had a sweet tooth and helped themselves to sugars if they had a chance. This was of little consequence with our sugar for morning teabreak, but the pure quality of analytical-grade glucose, for instance, was not improved by dirty hands used to scoop it out and shovel it into the mouth. All bottles of sugar reagents were treated as if they were scheduled drugs and kept in a locked cabinet.

Amongst the junior staff were several with whom I had daily contact. Nayaba Vom, an important figure in the local village, had a responsible job in the virology laboratory. He always wore dark glasses, because for many years he sealed the glass ampoules of vaccines, many hundreds of thousands of them. After the primary freeze-drying, the ampoules were first constricted, then placed on the rubber nipples of the secondary freeze driers where they were later sealed with a very hot flame while under vacuum. We used Edwards primary and secondary freeze-driers, rows of them, because of the lower running costs, and any which broke down were cannibalised constantly to keep the remainder running.

Nayaba was for ever having trouble with his motor-scooter, and when repairs became necessary he looked upon me as a soft touch, until I got wise. Whenever I was approached by laboratory staff or houseboys for a loan, I only lent them small sums of money, interest-free, if the borrower had already saved half the total amount he wanted to borrow. If staff got into the clutches of the village money-lenders they never got out of debt.

Sale, an evil-looking rogue if ever there was one, looked after the washing up. Johnson Onovo, an Ibo, helped me a great deal when I was working with tissue cultures. For a brief period a girl, Theresa, worked with me, fluttering her eyelashes at me whenever I instructed her how to prepare reagents, until one day I had to break up a real shouting-match next door, and Nayaba Vom stormed up to me threatening to resign if 'that harlot' was not removed instantly.

Many of the ills besetting Nigeria were blamed on Tribalism. In spite of repeated attempts to break the infiltration of Ibos into the north, they still persisted in coming, given the chance. Expatriate staff in the laboratory and our administrative branch received strict instructions that if a junior job vacancy could be filled by a northerner, then he must be appointed. If an Ibo Chief Clerk was allowed to make the appointment, invariably one of his remote relations, several times removed, would get the job.

Signs of dissension were already apparent and civil unrest seemed not far below the surface A general strike was called by the workers' unions in Lagos and because of the threat of sabotage to essential services around the laboratory and farm by dissident junior staff, the senior staff, particularly the few remaining expatriate staff amongst them, were briefed as to their duties. Water supplies and emergency electric generators were high on the list of items to be protected, though I am still not sure how I would have reacted, if confronted by an angry mob waving sticks. We were all highly amused when told why an earlier strike failed up north. Apparently workers in some post offices in the north, Vom was one, failed to distribute telegrams to unions in their vicinity before going on strike themselves. On another occasion while I was on leave, the army had been called in to protect essential services. I heard that a machine-gunner, sending a stream of tracer bullets into the far distance, had dispelled any further thought of action amongst the strikers.

By the wet season of 1965, Phase One of the Rinderpest campaign (JP15), which started in the countries around Lake Chad and included the northern provinces of Nigeria, had completed its third year. To get the maximum coverage of vaccination, every animal was supposed to have received a shot of rinderpest vaccine once a year for three years, so that if animals were missed in the first or second years, they would be done in the third − after all only one shot of vaccine was required to effectively immunise the animal. As proof of vaccination each animal received a clover-leaf punch mark on the ear each time they were vaccinated. By the end of Phase One, many of the older animals should have had three punch marks.

There were some misgivings that the system was being abused when animals only a year old were found with three punch marks. Naturally the funding organisations required some further proof that the vaccination campaign had been successful, and this could best be achieved by demonstrating the levels of rinderpest antibody in the cattle population.

Les Rowe, who was recruited from Britain to produce TCRV, had by this time produced adequate stocks for the estimated seven million cattle in the country. He was asked to carry out the antibody estimations. The veterinary staff in the north were supposed to collect serum samples from cattle all over the country, but with shortages of staff in the field the samples were slow to come in.

As our contribution to the overall effort, senior professional and technical staff from the laboratory in Vom were sent to the southern Plateau during the 1965 wet season to bleed cattle at a place called Bokkos. Our huge mobile laboratory, like an articulated caravan equipped with centrifuges and freezers powered by a diesel generator, was driven down and installed beside the Bokkos Rest House. We all went down for a week at a time to help the local veterinary assistants. Some of the staff were encouraged to take their wives and families too and make a bit of a holiday of it. The mobile laboratory was used to separate and store the serum, once the blood samples had been collected from the Fulani cattle.

In spite of a total lack of facilities for restraining cattle, no cattle crushes, nothing, samples were collected relatively easily. We started at dawn. The cattle, even the large bulls, were comparatively docile. It was the Fulani custom to hobble the adult beasts in pairs by their front legs at night. By putting casting ropes on each animal of a pair and pulling them one against the other, they invariably collapsed on the ground looking like one-armed wrestlers. I was constantly amazed they never broke a leg. Plenty of helpers then sat on the animals and the intrepid bleeder did his job with little fuss, taking a good blood sample from the jugular vein, though occasionally a rope would come undone prematurely and then it was everyone for himself.

We only aimed at about a thousand samples a week, so the pace was leisurely. By late morning each day we had done our quota, and the rest of the day was devoted to looking around the local scene. On one of our rambles near the resthouse we stumbled upon large white stones almost hidden in the grass, spelling in large letters the word BOKKOS, and thought we had found some strange native sacred site, until it dawned on me that the cleared area in front was an airstrip, long disused, probably prepared during the war as an emergency strip. At that time regular flights linked Egypt with West Africa and subsequently by sea to Britain, the only safe route available for military personnel from Egypt to Britain during the early part of the North African campaign.

The Bokkos birds were similar to those around Vom, except for several male Pin-tailed Whydahs which displayed in the long grass around where we bled the cattle, looking like animated black and white puppets as they bounced up and down.

With Dantiyi to minister to our needs and look after the cooking on the rather primitive wood stove, June and I enjoyed walking the dogs late each afternoon. Alas, Lassie had gone to the happy hunting grounds by this time and was no doubt chasing bustard, bushfowl and snipe over the Elysian horizon. However we now possessed a miniature poodle, Fifi, from an expatriate couple who had left the country for good. We were also looking after an enormous Bull Mastiff-Rhodesian Ridgeback cross, called Joe, owned by private miner, Neville Priestley, who was away on leave.

Joe was a very placid dog, but towards the end of our stay in Bokkos Fifi came on heat and we had the most entertaining trip back to Vom in our little Fiat 1100. June in the front passenger seat had Fifi under her feet, trying hard to defend her honour. Joe in the back left little room for Dantiyi, taking almost the whole seat. He should have been admiring the scenery, but I drove most of the way home with one hand, trying hard to stop him joining us in the front, in spite of Dantiyi hauling hard on his collar. Never mind the scenery, Joe seemed to say, let's get on with the game. With their enormous discrepancy in size I doubt they could have managed, but Joe was eager to prove me wrong.

Joe's size caused many exclamations of admiration from the Nigerians in Vom. One morning he provided some of the laboratory staff with a bit of entertainment to brighten their day. It certainly made mine.

Pet owners were encouraged to dip their dogs once a week in a stone bath of insecticide at the Veterinary School clinic, because ticks were quite a problem and they transmitted a blood parasite which caused Tick Fever. Lassie had got so accustomed to this weekly event that she would jump into the dip of her own accord, but Joe was far too large. Soon after Joe joined us, we decided the cattle spray race at the laboratory was the perfect answer. The first time we decided to try it, June brought Joe to the spray race just before breakfast one morning, walked him in and sat him down. Normally very obedient, Joe obviously suspected something and followed her out. June turned back with Joe just as I gave the nod to the head stockman, Yahaya Kano, to start the pump. Unable to see the spray race at the same time, Yahaya heard the laughter and reappeared from the pumphouse in time to see Joe beat June out of the spray by a wet whisker.

Yahaya Kano, tall and very strong, was always courteous but seemed a trifle haughty. I once saw him pit his strength against one of our dwarf Muturu bullocks. Four of these vicious ugly short-legged brutes were kept as serum donors for tissue culture medium and bled once a month, always a tussle, for they were very undisciplined and savage. One had kicked Yahaya so hard on the thigh I feared a broken bone at least, then had reared up and fell back on him, knocking him to the ground. He picked himself up, dusted himself down, then wrestled the beast to the ground, in much the same way a shepherd turns up a sheep and with little more effort. Yet when June emerged dripping from her involuntary shower on that memorable morning, Yahaya was dreadfully embarrassed, wringing his hands and apologising profusely, in spite of my laughed reassurances, *'Ba kome, shi ke nan'.*

The Laboratories of the Federal Department of Veterinary Research in Vom were quite a showpiece, which regularly attracted visits from V.I.P.s, who sometimes descended in droves. We were always warned of impending visits, so had time to lay out displays of our activities, but since the routine work of vaccine production had to proceed uninterrupted, much of this went on behind closed doors. However the internal corridors, along which the visitors were ushered, were lined with windows looking into the various rooms, which allowed them to see some of our techniques without jeopardising the sterility of the work or endangering the visitors.

Some Ministerial groups swept through with hardly a pause, with supercilious glances, as if they knew it all, and hardly a word of encouragement for the workers. Others seemed really interested in the work we were doing, pausing, asking questions and taking their time. A spider's web full of spiderlings, inadvertently left in the corner of a newly-constructed sterile hood, which was displayed prominently on a bench as a means of minimising bacterial contamination, evoked the comment from one rather jovial Minister, 'I say, that spider doesn't look very sterile.' Once I even managed to give the Northern Nigerian Governor quite

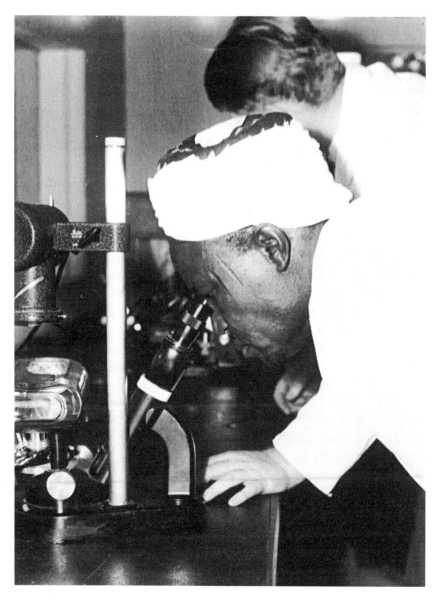

Governor of Northern Nigeria looking at tissue cultures. Vom 1964

a dissertation on the merits of the new tissue-cultured Rinderpest Vaccine.

Several overseas visitors also descended on us about this time and we were generally pleased to see them, especially if we shared common interests. Early in 1965 I corresponded with an American dentist, Larry Walkinshaw, also an ornithologist who devoted his spare time to studying the cranes of the world. In his first letter he asked me whether it was possible to get up to Lake Chad during the wet season to study the breeding of the West African Crowned Crane. Remembering my experiences in that area at the end of my first tour – barrier passes, four-wheel drive and mud galore – on our way to Gashua, I replied advising him against going up there at that time of year, but suggested that he would not lack suitable study subjects on the Plateau.

Larry arrived by air in July, stayed with us for a month, and was not disappointed with what he found around Vom. Most mornings he disappeared at dawn on foot and we had to send Badung out to find him with sandwiches and coffee. Badung put up a grass matting hide on one nest near the house, which pleased Larry no end. He took a lot of photographs and made many observations. Some years later, after we left Nigeria, we were delighted to receive a complimentary copy of his book, *Cranes of the World*, but rather embarrassed that the chapter on the West African Crowned Crane had almost as much to say about the Smith family as the birds themselves.

From the United States we had several visiting scientists. It seemed to me that they were all keen to investigate whether their money, in the form of USAID poured in to Nigeria for various internationally-funded projects, had been well spent. Within the space of a few months a group from the American Academy of Science, a party from their Virus Research Institute at Plum Island and a couple from their Communicable Diseases Centre all descended on us. Their interests, professional and otherwise, ranged over a wide variety of subjects and they all had to be entertained, which put a bit of a strain on our household resources, for we did not receive any entertainment allowance. One gentleman from Montana, who liked to look at minerals in

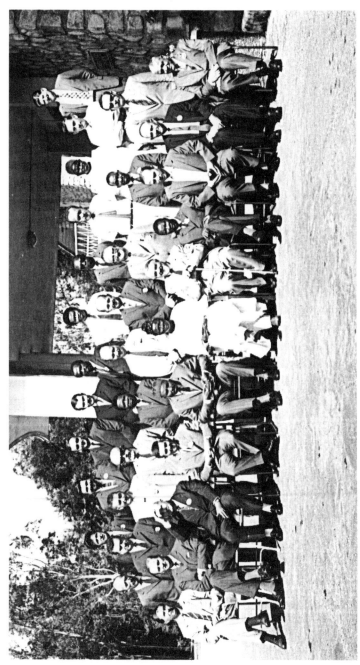

Delegates at JP15 Conference in Vom, 1965

countries he visited, decimated my carefully collected samples of tin ore.

Strangest of all were the Russians. We enjoyed the company of a party of Soviet scientists who visited Vom, accompanied by Alex Fedorov, Second Secretary to the Soviet Embassy. The purpose of their visit to Nigeria was ostensibly to investigate a source of live monkeys for research, so they travelled around the country and even visited Yankari Game Reserve where they later made themselves very unpopular by shooting some green monkeys.

Their leader, Professor Lapin, a former wartime pilot and hero, hobbled around very capably on his artificial legs and although only some spoke English and a couple no English at all, they were easy to entertain and generous with their gifts. At a lunch party we held for them, June invited the only lady member of their team to dish out the sweet, a very tasty apple pie prepared by Dantiyi to June's recipe. Our lady guest divided the pie meticulously into eight absolutely equal portions with much debate amongst her five colleagues We were rather amused, but taken aback by the several cartons of Russian cigarettes, strong and rank, which they pressed on us when taking their leave. I little realised at the time how useful I would find the cigarettes later. Their next visit to Nigeria was ill-timed as they arrived about the time of the military coup. They had some fast talking to do when they were stopped and searched at a military road-block, for the boot of their car was filled with an assortment of hunting rifles.

A Bovine Pleuropneumonia expert from C.S.I.R.O. in Australia, Len Lloyd, spent a few days studying our technique for preparing the Bovine Pleuropneumonia vaccine and blood-testing for reactors. Eager to meet anyone from a country which might offer future job opportunities, we entertained him and I picked his brains on life in Australia, little realising that within a year or so I would be enjoying life in that country.

CHAPTER 8

Last Vom Tour
and Many Migrant Birds

I HAD DECIDED THIS WOULD BE MY LAST TOUR and gave the required year's notice in September, to leave in March 1966. I had already accrued six months deferred leave. Two promising Nigerian veterinarians had by this time joined the Virology Division, Mba Uzoukwu and Kelsey Benibo David-West. I wanted to leave my Nigerian successor in the Virology Division, whoever he might be, with adequate stocks of all vaccines.

Although TCRV had come out a real winner in the JP15 campaign and several tested batches were in hand, I decided to leave good stocks of DGV also. We provided vaccines for all the former British Colonies and territories in West Africa, Gambia, Sierra Leone and Ghana (formerly Gold Coast) but also had to supply rinderpest vaccines for later phases of JP15. I was concerned that there might be problems with TCRV production in the future.

The success of the JP15 campaign in our immediate vicinity had already caused one problem in the laboratory. The rinderpest vaccines required unvaccinated animals free of antibodies in which vaccine batches could be tested. Supplies of antibody-free serum were also required as an ingredient of the growth medium for the cell cultures in which TCRV was grown. Such donor animals were becoming increasingly difficult to purchase locally, because all cattle over six months of age had to be vaccinated. It was because of this that we had purchased four Muturu cattle from the south. These ugly dwarf cattle were not even considered to be cattle by northerners. In spite of their cantankerous nature, their serum promoted good growth of tissue cultures. These animals were, of course, unvaccinated and held in strict isolation.

For testing batches of vaccine we purchased Fulani Zebu animals at six months of age and kept them also in isolation until they lost their maternal antibodies, the passive immunity conferred on them through their mother's milk. Les Rowe and Vivien Oreffo determined this by examining blood samples from these calves at monthly intervals.

The levels of maternal antibody in calves were a reflection of their mothers' level of antibodies. Some calves from mothers with high antibody levels possessed maternal antibodies until they were ten months of age, which interfered with their vaccination. Much of the research in which we were engaged revolved around improving techniques for vaccine production or in investigating and attempting to solve such problems. While I studied this interesting phenomenon of maternal protection in calves, Dik Zwart, Ian Macadam and Les Rowe tackled an equally vexing problem and studied the effects of rinderpest virus in smaller ruminants, like sheep and goats, in which French research scientists had already demonstrated a rinderpest-like disease called *Peste de petit ruminants* (PPR). During their studies they also encountered other strange viruses of cattle not previously recorded in Nigeria, like IBR from the urine of some of their in-contact cattle.

To minimise the number of animals required for testing each batch of vaccine, I increased each batch size of DGV by using a larger number of goats, and decided to order 200 goats a week, instead of 160. Out of 200 perhaps 140 would be suitable. I found a source of larger goats also and at the same time learnt how bribery played such an important part in the African logic.

The true meaning of the custom of 'Dash' was brought home to me, when June telephoned me one morning, greatly excited, and asked me to return home immediately. Not sure whether to expect some domestic disaster, or perhaps some rare bird in the mist-net, I was astonished to find my garage full of vegetable produce, including sacks of potatoes. A number of live fowls with legs tied together garnished the whole pile.

Dantiyi could only tell me they had been left by one of the contractors, whose name he had conveniently forgotten. It was renewal-of-goat-contract time and I usually chose the regular contractor, but this year there was another contender who promised larger goats. How could I refuse, though I am still not sure whose vegetable produce filled my garage. Each of the new goats provided about 5000 cattle doses so our production target was over half a million doses a week continuously over several weeks.

DGV was a remarkably simple vaccine to produce as it utilised the junior staff to their maximum ability. There were, however, limitations to production. It had been found in the past that if DGV preparation was attempted during the wet season, the newly-delivered goats rapidly died from various respiratory diseases probably provoked by their transport to the colder Plateau altitude. Thus it was necessary to wait for the 1965 dry season before commencing my last onslaught on DGV production.

Goats were received on Fridays and their temperatures taken daily over the weekend by junior staff. On Monday morning goats with normal temperatures were inoculated with the seed virus and their temperatures taken daily till the end of the week. Friday was the big day, and the aim was to get the tissues from the goats into the primary freeze-dryers by breakfast time. We commenced about 5.00 a.m. when junior staff started to take the goat temperatures. Their temperature on the Friday morning was all important as it indicated which animals had reacted satisfactorily to the seed virus. A senior officer selected those goats which were suitable and these were run through first. They were shot with a humane killer and their spleens removed and placed in a chilled container. The pulp from each spleen was homogenised in a chilled colloid mill and put into bulk containers which were then placed in the freeze-dryers.

The whole business was noisy and smelly. Goats bleating – goat numbers being shouted out – temperatures called – muted shots – Bang! – and an overall sickly odour of blood pervaded by the smell of the goats. The rejected goats were killed as soon as the others had been run through and all the carcases had to be disposed of and the whole place washed down and thoroughly disinfected before the next batch of goats arrived later in the morning. The tight schedule worked well as long as nothing went wrong.

Caprinised Rinderpest Virus was not infectious for humans, in fact in the past many Veterinary Officers in the field were tempted to eat rinderpest-infected meat because the associated fever tenderised the rather tough local beef. Consequently all goat carcases were sold to the African staff. Each goat cost us two pounds but the staff paid only five shillings each for the carcases so got excellent value. It was a practical way of increasing their protein intake as meat was generally too expensive for them. And bearing in mind the close relationship between rinderpest and measles viruses, who knows but the goat virus may have protected the African children from measles, though we never had the opportunity to work on this interesting subject.

The skin of the goats made fine Morocco leather and to recoup some of our financial loss the Principal Executive Officer once suggested the carcases should be skinned before sale to the junior staff. What an indignant response that suggestion provoked! So the staff continued to get their carcases complete and were able to recover their outlay by selling the skins, thus getting an abundant feast of meat free.

The most vivid memory I have of Fridays when DGV production was in full swing was returning to my house for breakfast, feeling I had done a full days work, past an endless line of goat carcases being carried to the junior staff quarters. There were carcases in wheelbarrows – carcases draped across bicycles – and invariably carcases in the ubiquitous headpans with the little toto underneath almost overwhelmed by goat legs dangling down on all sides. Yet always they grinned the inevitable greeting – 'Sannu Bature'.

The homogenised spleen pulp remained on the primary freeze-driers overnight. On the Saturday morning the dried powder was measured into bottles and stored in bulk, a far less tedious business than sealing glass ampoules over a weekend. All the other vaccines were sealed by Nayaba Vom off the secondary freeze-driers on the second day after harvesting, and that was a very labour-consuming business. Thus planning DGV production for a Friday ensured that the freeze-drying machines were utilised throughout the week to their practical limit.

Each vaccine batch was tested at different dilutions in susceptible cattle, some of which were later challenged with a large dose of an earlier proven batch of DGV. The younger animals we were later compelled to use often reacted severely with a rather alarming blood-stained diarrhoea. In addition to causing a fever, the vaccine inflamed the bowel sometimes stirring up latent coccidial infections, a condition in calves which fortunately responded to an intravenous injection of sulphamezathine. I found it was quite an anxious time testing vaccine batches and the calves were not the only ones to undergo psychological trauma.

To provide an escape from pressure of work, I got involved in several extra-mural activities about this time. During my last year I became the Secretary of the Rayfield Sailing Club, a seemingly ostentatious title for a group of enthusiasts and their families who derived a lot of pleasure messing about in boats on one of the mining dams near Barakin Ladi. What about schistosomiasis, we asked ourselves. Just before the Sailing Club moved to this dam we were visited in Vom by a scientist, a snail expert, who looked carefully around the edges of the dam and found none of the snails which act as an intermediate host for this parasite. Without the snail there could be no risk of infection to us, perhaps as well, because some of us novice sailors spent almost as much time in the water as on it.

The Sailing Club was but one of the many facilities encouraged by the big mining company on the Plateau, the Amalgamated Tin Mines of Nigeria (ATMN), who provided the little aluminium sailing dinghies. I cannot even remember their name or design, but they had tripod masts and were gaff-rigged and were simple to sail single-handed though there was room for two.

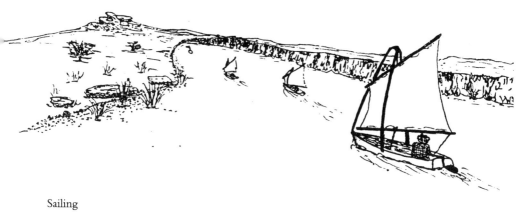

Sailing

The club even boasted a club-house made of cement blocks at the water's edge and a rescue boat, much in demand as the winds were fluky and an unexpected gybe sometimes tipped dinghies over. Their built-in buoyancy stopped them from sinking, but assistance was required to right them.

We had a regatta or two, when we were visited by members from other clubs who were always far too polite to laugh at our meagre resources. Our members, however, found the resources adequate and the facilities ideal for spending a pleasurable Sunday afternoon on the water. My most painful duty as Secretary was to write a letter of condolences to the wife of an expatriate, not a club member, who tried his hand at sailing when no one else was about, capsized and drowned. The dam was very deep in places.

The ATMN Clubs were open to their senior Nigerian staff, yet few seemed to become members. Perhaps Clubs were too much an English institution, or maybe they could not afford the subscriptions. By contrast our Vom Club was open to all senior laboratory staff and by 1965 many Nigerians had attained senior professional or technical status. It was a popular meeting place on Saturdays at the end of the week's work, and we sometimes organised afternoon children's sports of the light-hearted kind on the tennis court, not big enough for sprints and jumping, yet ample for three-legged, egg-and-spoon and wheelbar-row races.

As Chairman of the Club Committee during my last tour, I was one of only two expatriates on the Committee. By this time much of the talent of our former Amateur Dramatic Society had left, so few plays and shows were put on during my last year. I remember one of the functions we put on during my tenure, more for the events which subsequently followed. Our pride-and-joy, a newly installed cash register, was missing the following morning. It contained no money but the repercussions reverberated around Vom, as claims and counter-claims were made about the possible 'Teefman.' In disgust I eventually resigned as Chairman when one of the Committee members claimed she had heard voices in the night telling her who the criminal was.

I suspect that a club member living nearby had removed and hidden the cash register to make a point without any malicious intent, when he found that the Bar Secretary who was always last out, had forgotten to lock the Club door after the function. When the police were called in he probably felt he should keep quiet about his involvement in the whole business.

In spite of these other activities, I had by this time made a lot of interesting observations on the breeding habits of many of the local birds, much of it already written up during the long evenings in articles which had been published in *The Nigerian Field*, illustrated in some cases with photographs kindly offered to me by other enthusiasts. I had also accu-mulated amongst my reels of colour film, some sequences of some of the rarer birds at their nests, so had put together a number of short films which I showed at Nigerian Field Society meetings in Jos and on visits to Zaria and Kano, where I also spoke briefly on the control of animal diseases in Nigeria, thereby justifying a legitimate claim for travelling expenses.

I had also looked at possible illness in migrant birds, admittedly not for viral diseases which would have been too hard with our limited resources, but for blood parasites. A scientist from Kings College in London, who visited us in Vom, had already asked me to prepare blood films from any migrant birds I caught, offering to examine them for me. This I was able to do during my last tour. All I had to do was take a minute drop of blood from the toe of each individual bird and prepare a thin blood film on a glass microscope slide, which I then identified by the bird's ring number scratched on with a diamond pencil. After fixing each smear with alcohol, I sent the slides, some three hundred altogether, to Frank Cox in batches.

It was some years later that I received his final report, by which time I was in Australia and had already published in *Ibis* a paper on the spring and autumn weights of the various species of migrants I had caught in Vom. He had found some of my birds parasitised with two blood parasites, namely a *Haemaproteus* species, which is generally supposed to be harmless, and a *Plasmodium* species, a form of bird malaria of the same group of organisms which caused human malaria. The infections seemed to be picked up by the birds soon after they arrived in West Africa, but did not seem to cause them any inconvenience. It was almost as if the migrant birds had become accustomed to such infections, which could well be the case because this form of long distance bird migration between Africa and Europe has been going on for a very long time. West Africa became 'The White Man's Grave' only through white men's lack of previous exposure to the disease organisms and seemed to have no equivalent in the bird world.

I was determined to make our last dry season a memorable one with regard to bird ringing. Yellow wagtails were one species of migrant bird on which we were able to concentrate our resources. From early days I had noticed that during the dry season they were usually seen in small groups feeding on the insects disturbed by native Fulani cattle as they grazed all around Vom and even down at Bokkos. I knew wagtails roosted communally, because in the early 1960s Bob Sharland had started to catch them using mist-nets at a roost in Kano about 200 miles north of Vom.

His roost was in reeds in one of the borrow-pits from which soil had been excavated to make the earthen walls and mud buildings of the old Kano city. The borrow-pits were most insalubrious, for they soon turned into cess-pits, full of filthy water, into which all the rubbish was thrown and the effluent of the native city drained. Bob urged me to find a roost on the Plateau in more healthy surroundings.

Not long after Bob's impassioned plea, I was sitting near a mining dam late one afternoon with Dave Ebbutt, a keen ornithologist working at the Government Trade Centre near Vom. We saw a small group of wagtails fly over obviously on their way to roost, so took a bearing on their flight line. Later we took bearings on other flocks going to roost and plotted them on a map. Tracks seemed to converge over a eucalyptus plantation. These imported trees grew well on the Plateau, and provided firewood and poles for native huts, but the plantations were rather sterile of bird-life and we seldom walked through them.

On this occasion, however, we investigated one evening at dusk and

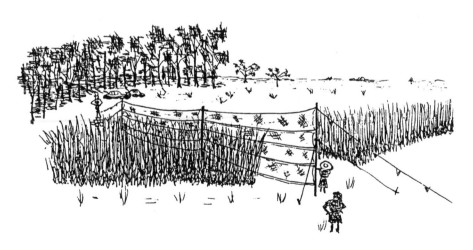

Netting Yellow Wagtails in a swamp

found a swamp in the centre of the plantation in which large numbers of wagtails – many thousands – were roosting. We watched, quite fascinated, until it was almost too dark to see and realised it would require a major operation to try and net them, but not entirely devoid of possibility. One fact in our favour was that this plantation was only two miles from my house and even closer to Dave's.

The birds started to come in about an hour before dusk. They flew around high before dropping almost vertically, undoubtedly to avoid predation, because we often saw falcons circling over the roost. Mist-nets would not catch many when they arrived, of that we were sure. However by putting the nets up before dusk and then having a beat or two, we found the birds flew along just over the tops of the tall swamp grass.

Garden boy Badung was promised a handsome reward if he cut a swathe through the centre of the swamp, which by this time of the year was quite dry underfoot. He did this without complaint, though we discovered later that the six-foot high swamp grass was covered in little barbs which led to intense itchiness. Forestry officer Mike Horwood allowed us to thin out three straight eucalyptus saplings about twenty feet high, which we planted upright in the swathe. On these we were able to raise two long mist-nets on poles to a level just above the top of the swamp grass, on pulleys so that they could be later lowered to remove any birds. It was a crudely improvised system but worked.

The swamp burnt down soon after we found the first roost, but by our most astonishing good fortune the birds moved into a patch of sugar-cane, only a few hundred metres from the front of my house. Besides providing a much cleaner environment, it was so much easier to approach and we always gave the owner a few bob for his approval. By this time I had also started to use ten foot lengths of gas piping on which to support the nets.

Our first catches were fortunately small. We soon realised that to cope with larger numbers of birds before total darkness descended on us, we would have to recruit a lot of help. June suggested we invite some of the families in Vom for afternoon tea, after which we would sally forth to catch wagtails with all the recruits we wanted. She also suggested that instead of ringing birds in the dark at the swamp, where the mosquitoes were almost as large and abundant as the wagtails, we should bring the birds home and ring them in the comfort of the lounge. Later, because birds released in the dark tended to fly into lighted windows, we then decided to hold them overnight and let them go at dawn.

So it was, from the 1963 dry season onwards, we provided light evening entertainment for quite a few of our friends. Amongst the regular attenders were the Ebbutts, Godfreys, Woods, Langs, Grays, Roberts and Mike Horwood. Mike, after years of camping out in the bush as a Forestry Officer, was always good for regaling us with an account of how to build a B.G. in the bush, though I could never fathom what this had to do with wagtails.

Fortified with chocolate cake, as only June could make, we sallied forth an hour before dusk and got the nets up in good time. The birds rarely got tangled badly. The wives with their nimble fingers frantically extricated the birds from the nets. Placed in cardboard beer cartons with sleeves of old shirts sewn in at one end for easy access, the birds were taken back to the house where they were ringed, measured and weighed and suffered other indignities. Later June improved the social side of things by providing supper too, generally Spaghetti Bolognese, for the helpers, that is, not the wagtails.

The numerous beer cartons used for holding the birds overnight were generally suitable provided the birds were not crowded. At the height of the dry season during our first wagtail year, when the birds were moulting and at their lowest weight, I was distressed when we found some birds dead in the boxes after an oppressive night. From then on the beer cartons were only used for transporting birds to the house. Once ringed and measured they spent the night in a large dog kennel, the same one in which Lassie had accompanied me to Nigeria. This worked admirably and on mornings after, at dawn, a veritable cloud of wagtails would fly off. Few birds died after that.

One evening we caught about 330 birds, our biggest nightly catch. We ringed nearly twelve thousand during several seasons. David and I made some useful contributions to the knowledge of their moult, measurements, weights and sub-specific differences, which we published in an earlier article in *Ibis*. Up to the time I left Nigeria, several recoveries were reported to us, the most notable being a bird recovered north of Leningrad. Many of our birds were recaptured during subsequent seasons, showing considerable fidelity to their winter haunts. Some birds we caught bore Kano rings and Bob reported at least one of our birds turning up there. Wagtails bearing Italian rings and with the return address *Moskwa* gave us our greatest thrill.

Once, a heavy afternoon thunderstorm stopped us going out at dusk. The oppressive humidity late in March made me call off the party and instead I was writing letters when our house received a spectacular direct hit, the tin roof amplifying the thunder which was deafening. The old bakelite telephone beside me exploded – 'Finished please? – Finished? -Finished?' Indeed! An electric fire against the wall threw out huge sparks. Later when the torrential rain stopped, mainly to settle my frayed nerves which were still twanging like guitar strings, David and I went out to the sugar cane after dark with torches to see what effect the storm might have had on the birds. They seemed stupefied and by hand we managed to catch nearly a hundred.

The daily dispersal of these wagtails intrigued us, particularly how far they went from the roost. The shiny aluminium rings on their legs were rarely visible, even in the shortest grass when the birds were amongst cattle, so we decided to mark some. White on their outer tail feathers showed plainly as the birds spread their tails when landing, so we dipped their tails in picric acid in alcohol. It did them no harm, but this yellow dye turned orange later and was quite conspicuous. Although we colour-marked some five hundred birds, we only saw one later in the field.

Every pack has a joker, and one evening our court jester rose to the occasion most appropriately. 'Wouldn't we get more spectacular results colour-marking the white Cattle Egrets?' he facetiously suggested. 'You know, the ones which roost in that tree near the Vet Clinic? With a stirrup pump after dark – bucketfuls of histological stains – we could do some blue one night – some red the next – add a really patriotic touch to our efforts.' Pressure of other work fortunately prevented us from trying this.

We gathered a lot of interesting information on other species of birds. During the height of one dry season, we caught a number of small birds which we later identified as cuckoo weavers, about which little was known except that they parasitised other weavers. Hil Fry was up from Zaria on that occasion and we prepared some skin specimens for the British Museum.

I seemed to become the butt of any light-hearted humour during these evenings. I was once asked to examine an unidentified bird in one of the catching boxes and without a thought thrust my hand into the sleeve. I at first thought someone with a perverted sense of humour had put a snake in the carton, as an irate Red-necked Falcon sank its needle-sharp claws into my fingers. This dashing little bird of prey, chasing wagtails over the sugar-cane, had finished up in the net itself much to its annoyance.

In moments of high excitement in the field, tempers got very brittle and during my last tour I must have been the chief offender, drawing freely on my extensive vocabulary of barrackroom phrases. That no one left in disgust constantly amazed me. However, as the end of my last season approached, our court jester and wit did tackle me one evening. He was sure that some of my more explicit phrases would complement the Glossary of Wagtailing Terms he was compiling, but he was not sure what they meant or how they would translate into Hausa.

I made my first and only appearance in a Nigerian court, and at the same time learnt what it was like to be without a car, only a few months before my final departure. One Sunday, while looking forward to a curry lunch in Yelwa Club after a session filming birds at Kafo Rock, I was driving to Bukuru with June, fortunately not at my usual breakneck speed, when I hit an elderly Birom gentleman. The stupid idiot, absolutely befuddled with drink, ran across in front of me. In turn I swerved to the wrong side of the road and did my little Fiat 1100 a lot of injury when I hit the parapet of a bridge culvert concealed in the long grass. The Birom's two sons were taking their drunk father home after an all-night binge on the locally-brewed atcha beer and turned out to be good witnesses on my behalf.

However about three weeks later the police charged me with dangerous driving causing an accident. Lots of advice came my way from colleagues and friends in Vom, some rather coarse with little sympathy, but most important of all I was told to mention the matter to our Principal Executive Officer, Mallam Mayo, who immediately offered to have a word with the police. My case came up in the native Alkhali's court and I was a bit upset when an expatriate solicitor in Jos refused to represent me but found an African for me. Very wisely I realised later, for only African legal eagles were present in the court presided over by a Pakistani magistrate. The case was dismissed in five minutes, but the magistrate spent another five minutes moralising about the high number of accidents caused by expatriates – I was delighted when my African solicitor caught my eye and said afterwards, 'What a load of twaddle.'

I was more fortunate than a young lady from Vom Mission who accidentally killed a mentally defective Nigerian in Jos Market. She had to back her car out from a narrow lane, not realising that the idiot had lain down on the road behind her. Her companion whisked her away in a highly distraught state and she was flown out of the country within twenty-four hours on medical grounds. The possibility of accidents on the road was, I am sure, in most people's minds, especially when driving out in the bush. Had anyone been unfortunate enough to injure an African, say while driving through a remote village, their best course of action was to drive on to the next village before reporting it to the police, rather than face a hostile crowd.

Several families left in late 1965, amongst them the Thornes. Tony was

Director from 1960 and Deputy Director before that. Emmanuel Eze-buiro, an Ibo, was promoted from Deputy Director to become Acting Director. I had already decided to leave in March 1966, so expressed little interest in the Deputy post, not that I was pressed to take it anyway, though I suppose I could have contested it on seniority.

During my last tour I thought a lot about the Sahara Desert. The French still had a military presence in Algeria and were in the habit of letting off atomic bombs at their two testing sites. Considerable concern had been expressed about radio-active fall-out in Nigeria, brought south-wards by the *Harmattan*, though I believe nothing of significance was ever demonstrated by the monitoring. Nevertheless, I wondered about the many million migrant birds which crossed this huge desert twice a year. I was familiar with many of them in Scotland, also here in Nigeria, but what of the bit in between? What other hazards did the birds face? That they had been doing this twice yearly migration for countless years still did not ameliorate the difficulties encountered by them.

Reg Moreau had published an interesting double article in *Ibis* in 1962 discussing the physical problems encountered by these migrant birds and he first postulated the theory of migration on a broad front. I thought by motoring across during the spring northward movement, with ample time to make observations, I would see firsthand something of this migration. March seemed as good a time as any to depart, so mid-tour I started a sort of feasibility study. If I allowed two months for the whole trip back to Britain, what problems would I face.

My initial plans were to send June home by more conventional means and do the trip with a pen-pal from the Sudan, also interested in Trans-Saharan bird migration, who would join me in Kano. He backed out only three months or so before my intended departure, leaving me with no choice but to invite June who accepted, not without some misgivings. Roger would be at boarding school in Britain and was to spend his Easter holidays with his uncle and aunt in Shrewsbury.

The Australian manager of Plateau Dairy, Doug Woosley, offered to sell me their old Forward Control Land Rover, due to be traded in for a new model, so I had a good look at it. Such a vehicle would save me some embarassment. Originally I had rather fancifully contemplated doing the trip in my little Fiat 1100 – sturdy little car it was, but not really suitable for such a journey. The four-wheel drive, low ratio gearbox and large tyres of the Land Rover were to prove themselves a real boon in soft sand. The spacious vehicle allowed us to carry large reserves of water, food and fuel. In the back there was ample space for our large double bedding roll, a metal trunk which my father had carted all round India, all my bird-netting gear including ten foot lengths of gas piping suspended from the frame, two forty-four gallon drums of fuel and a twelve gallon drum of water, our precious reserve.

Not realising that in the desert there would be few observers of our daily evacuations and not enamoured with the crude 'Shave-on-a-shovel' favoured by the army during the desert war, or for that matter Mike Horwood's model of a bush B.G., I built ourselves an elaborate throne and June an enormous wigwam to sit over it, which we laughingly left in the middle of the Sahara, as we hardly ever needed the privacy it provided.

Since we would travel through former French territories, I was advised to contact the Paris Museum who co-ordinated the French Ringing Scheme. Not only did I receive a large supply of rings engraved with the return address *Museum Paris*, they also sent me a letter of introduction, which proved useful on more than one occasion, and gave me the name of a contact, André Dupuy, who would be working near Beni Abbes about the time I expected to pass through.

We were overwhelmed with offers of help and cast-off bits and pieces of camping gear. The Maintenance Superintendent in our workshop, Jack Dale, offered to check the vehicle thoroughly and fit racks on the sides. On one side were fitted racks for gerry cans. On the other, just behind the driver, he designed an ingenious compartment with drop-down shelf on which we could brew up. We did all our cooking on a primus and a couple of gallons of kerosene lasted us the whole six weeks. Jack also advised me on the formidable list of spare-parts I should take. He arranged to have the bulkier items, like spare springs and half-shafts, bolted on to the chassis or the bumper bars. By Christmas-time the whole exercise was beginning to look very promising.

We were determined to make our last Christmas in Vom a memorable and traditional one. With the usual warm dry days to be expected at this time of year in Vom, it was little wonder our thoughts generally tended to dwell on Christmas cards showing snow, frost, holly and robins. These were all incomprehensible to Nigerians. At an interview board for Nigerians hoping to further their training in Britain, I once showed a candidate a photograph of a picturesque snow scene and was surprised at his reaction. He could not grasp the fact that the snow did not fall in one solid lump.

June organised all the traditional Christmas fare – ham from the farm, turkey, plum-pudding and trimmings – and we invited a houseful of friends for lunch. After the meal we trooped outside to see the village children do their little charade, all dressed up in strange clothing, including one – 'The Red Funny Man' – who was symbolic of something, we

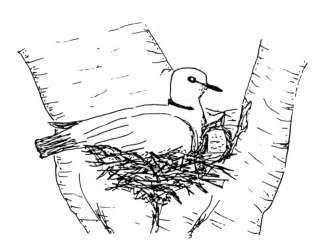

Vinaceous Turtle Dove on nest

were never quite sure what, though there seemed little of the Nativity about it.

Our seasonal festivities extended over several days and we held our customary drinks party on the morning of New Year's Day when we usually made up Pimms by the bucketful, looking more like a fruit salad, and dispensed tankards of it with largesse to all and sundry. It was certainly a very merry period.

Roger, out for his last holidays in Nigeria, was in on several parties. He was invited to the Vom Club Christmas Party and the Yelwa Club Christmas Party and somehow we fitted in his birthday party on the 28th December, to which most of the Vom senior staff children of his age were invited. For the first time the Nigerian kids outnumbered the expatriate ones.

Roger was due to return to school in Britain in mid-January. His return flight was on a Sunday and I was expected to make a quick trip by air to Lagos on the following day to interview staff. With still two months before our intended departure, I was sure I could fit it in.

It was Rabbie Burns, the Scottish Bard revered by Caledonian Society members, who said,

> 'The best laid schemes o' mice and men,
> Gang aft agley.'

CHAPTER 9

1966 Military Coup and
Departure Trans-Sahara

NIGERIA'S FIRST MILITARY COUP D'ETAT caught all of us in Vom totally
by surprise. On the Friday night just after the Commonwealth Prime
Ministers' Conference had concluded in Lagos and two days before
Roger was due to fly back to school for the last time, the military took
over. Ramadan was still on and the Hausa, never at their best during
this month-long Moslem fast, were stunned. Little work was done on
that Saturday morning as we stood around in little huddled groups and
discussed the news.

Confused radio broadcasts told us that a couple of Premiers had been
assassinated. One of them was the Sardauna of Sokoto, Sir Ahmadu
Bello, the spiritual leader and Premier of the Northern Region. The
other was Chief Akintola of the Western Region. We learnt later that
a number of high ranking army officers, mostly Northerners, were killed
in Lagos, amongst them a Birom, Colonel Pam.

Federal Prime Minister Sir Abubakar Tafawa Balewa, a man of great
integrity, honoured and admired, had been seized and was missing. The
Federal Finance Minister, Chief Samuel Festus Okotie-Eboh, less highly
regarded, corrupt and known as Festering Sam, was also missing but
both were later found murdered.

We got the impression in Vom that the coup was conceived by a
group of middle-cadre army officers, most of them Ibo. Of course it
had been well organised – Sandhurst-trained, all of them were. Apparently
night army exercises were conducted for several weeks around the
Sardauna's house in Kaduna, before that fateful Friday night when the
army dropped a mortar bomb through the roof and shot him at his door

as he came out to see what all the fuss was about. One of his wives tried to protect him and was also killed, as were all his bodyguards.

Relatively isolated as we were in Vom, we were all convinced a veritable blood-bath was in progress in the south of the country and elsewhere, so naturally I was most reluctant to go down to Lagos two days later. We solved the problem of what to do about Roger by keeping him with us so he got an extra weeks holiday, but the failure of overseas communications meant we were unable to let the school know what was going on.

Acting Director in Vom, Emmanuel Ezebuiro, wanted to know as much as anyone else what the situation was like in the Federal Capital. It took a lot of persuasion from him, perhaps prompted slightly by my natural morbid curiosity, before I agreed to fly down to Lagos on the Monday. Stepping off the Fokker Friendship into the high and unpleasant Lagos humidity, I was pleasantly surprised to find the situation there fairly normal. I heard later that a number of army officers had been shot on the golf course, not so strange a place to find their corpses, because their officers' mess backed on to it. At the airport there was no harassment, but I found it a bit disconcerting to see armed troops at Ikeja airport nonchalantly pointing their automatic weapons at navel height. At the airport I posted a letter home which I had scribbled on the plane and also sent a brief cable for good measure from the Cable Office.

The expatriates I spoke to in the bar of the Ikoyi Hotel in Lagos later that afternoon were surprised to learn I had come down from the north that day and stood me several beers. How had I avoided being massacred was the opening question. With each successive beer, no doubt my story improved. In fact, all round, there was little loss of life. I heard later that two expatriates who were killed had tried to force their way through a road block. The mass killings of the Ibos in the north came many months later.

My staff interviews completed, I stayed overnight in the Ikoyi Hotel, even though bloodstains were still visible on the floor where a senior army officer had been shot down. I could not get back to Vom fast enough and was already booked on the early morning return flight on the Tuesday. Ikeja airport being more than an hour's drive from Ikoyi, I arranged for departmental driver James Alabi to collect me in the darkness before dawn. Neither of us realised there was a curfew.

That night I believe someone had a go at General Ironsi, an Ibo, only recently recalled from the Congo where he had led the United Nations peace-keeping force. Whilst still in Ikoyi we drove slap-bang into an army roadblock in the dark, fortunately stopping just in time. The official-looking Land-Rover and my chalky-white face probably saved us from a blast of bullets. A gun barrel was thrust through the driver's side window and in the light of a torch shone on us, I noticed James had turned that pallid colour which looked almost sickly green with fear. I stuttered that we were on official business and tried to smile,

After what seemed an interminable time and was probably less than a minute, the owner of the gun barrel flashed his teeth in a wolfish grin, waved us on and I caught my plane. At Kaduna a group of army officers got off and I believe they were sent by General Ironsi to arrest − or perhaps offer safe conduct to − young Major Nzeiogwu, the Ibo who had led the coup in the north and killed the Sardauna. At Jos Airport June was so pleased to see me again, she burst into tears. Roger was more interested to know how many bodies had I seen.

Back on the Plateau, the seemingly rapid return to normal every day life was but an illusion, for the Hausa in the north were waiting their opportunity. Hausa executive officers with access to staff files were no doubt sifting through them to pick out the undesirable elements. Word was passed around from all kinds of sources that the coup had got rid of the unscrupulous elements in the Government, that it was a good thing, but I do not think anyone was deceived. It seemed too much of a good thing that many Northerners had been killed yet Ibos survived. Up to the time we departed in March there were no further troubles, but soon after we left, Ironsi himself was assassinated and the Hausa assumed control under General Gowon, a northern army officer who owed his life to being overseas in January.

Amongst those who helped us net wagtails was a geologist looking for diamond pipes in the north, Peter Woods. He and his wife Jenny were both keen bird-watchers. Not long before our intended date of departure, Peter insisted that I had a trial run with my newly acquired Land Rover and suggested a weekend trip down to the Fish Farm at Panyam, seventy miles or so south of Vom. Peter led me through some pretty rough terrain in his Landrover before we returned to Vom. I felt a lot more comfortable in my vehicle after that and more accustomed to the high driving position and absence of engine in front, for in this model the engine lay between driver and passenger. In the desert we appreciated the good view of the surface immediately in front and the relatively cool air which blew through the front vents.

Whilst making plans for the overland trip back to Britain I had also given the matter of my future employment some thought. I was of an age when new employment might not come easy. The question of Roger's schooling and a more settled family base also had to be considered. My options seemed a little limited. I could go back to Britain and perhaps apply for a job in the Ministry. I could try for an F. A. O. appointment somewhere in Africa. In fact about this time F. A. O. were seeking applicants for a Chief Research Officer post in Uganda. I applied but thought later how lucky I was not to get it, for the processing of my application took so long I had by then other irons in the fire. Perhaps it was as well, because if I had gone to Uganda I would have arrived there about the time Idi Amin came to power.

Two Australians in Vom, Doug Woosley who sold me the Landrover and Hal Hall, Principal of the Veterinary School, worked hard to persuade me to apply for a position in Western Australia where they had both worked in the past. The Chief Geologist with ATMN, Queenslander Tony Meehan, and an Australian dentist in Jos, Bill Thompson, also added their weight to the argument. I had by this time gained plenty of hands-on practical experience of several tropical diseases of domestic animals. Such diseases do not occur in Australia. I was perhaps fortunate that about the time of my departure from Nigeria the Australian authorities were looking for veterinary scientists with experience of such diseases.

In November I had written to the Chief of the Animal Health Laboratories in Perth offering my services.

During the few days prior to our motoring out of the front gate at Vom for the last time, we were kept fully occupied with many last minute details. Armed with the inevitable handing-over notes, I placed the Virology Division in the capable hands of K. B. David-West, little realising that soon afterwards he would go off on extended leave himself and never return to work in Vom. I had to almost plead for abnormal route allowances, not often granted on final departure. In return for its payment I was told I had to have a special medical to ensure I was fit to travel back to Britain by 'the overland route.'

Suitable homes were found for Fifi and Pyewacket. I found other employment for Dantiyi also, though I gave both him and Badung a sort of substantial terminal gratuity. I disposed of the Fiat, and some of my mist-netting equipment for the wagtails, just retaining enough to do a bit of netting on the way across the Sahara. Last of all, once I had despatched all our crates by rail to Lagos to go back to Britain by sea, we handed back the house to PWD and stayed with friends for the last couple of nights. And we attended numerous farewells . . .

So busy were we, we had little time to realise that we would soon be leaving what had been our home and garden for seven years and a Nigerian staff and place of work which still evoke many a happy memory. Yet our journey home, still to come, was also an exciting experience to look forward to and perhaps we might unravel a few more aspects of the intriguing problems of bird migration across the Sahara and tie up some of the ornithological loose ends we had unravelled on the Plateau.

Early in March, June and I departed Vom and set course northwards on

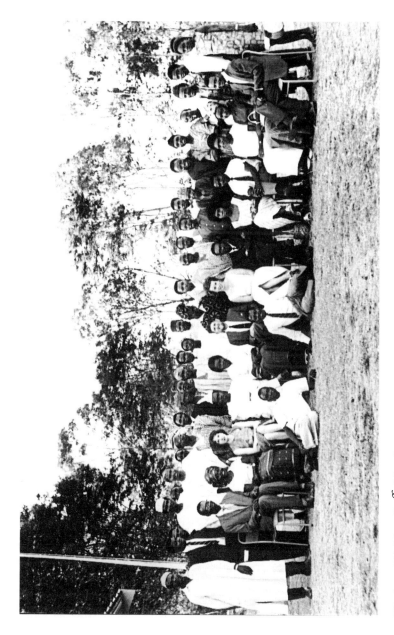

Virology Division Staff. March 1966

our six weeks journey back to Britain, excited about the unknown yet apprehensive, because the Sahara Desert is the largest in the world, larger than the whole land-mass of Australia where I hoped to go later the same year.

The Sahara shows great diversity. Huge sand-seas stretch hundreds of miles across the northern part, central volcanic massifs rise to over 10,000 feet, large areas of stony desert are so flat they allow one to drive very fast, occasional oases are scattered rather haphazardly like a few dozen cups set at random on a football field.

Two routes were suitable for vehicles. The western route started from Timbuktu, well west of Nigeria, and crossed the Tenezrouft, an immense area of featureless stony desert, offering few places where migratory birds might stop.

The eastern route went northwards from Kano through the centre of the northern border of Nigeria, passing over the Hoggar Massif in southern Algeria. Here surely would be some places suitable for studying the bird migration known to occur on such a vast scale. A Michelin map sent to us by the Automobile Association of Great Britain, showed a track joining the two routes across the Plain of Tidikelt, so we decided to start on the eastern route and then to cross to the western route later, as we were aiming for the Straits of Gibraltar.

We spent a leisurely few days in mid-March driving northwards. At Zaria we stayed with Hil Fry who visited us in Vom several times and was an authority on bee-eaters, particularly the Red-throated Bee-eater, which he had studied extensively. At Kano we stayed with the Sharlands, and I felt this augured well for the success of our migratory studies, because Bob had interested me in bird ringing.

It seemed to me from my netting experiences in Vom during several spring northward migrations, that the earlier birds would be starting across the Sahara about the third week in March, so I was optimistic that we would see some visible movement on the way if we left about the same time.

The day before departing from Kano we met a couple, the Sansoms, also travelling north in a long wheelbase Land Rover, so decided to travel together as far as Tamanrasset, where they would continue their journey while we spent a few days up in the mountains. We agreed to meet at the border post Daura at midday on the 24th March.

With petrol, water, provisions and bedding aboard, and several small personal items chained to the chassis as a deterrent against pilfering, our load was almost the maximum all-up weight permitted for the Forward Control Land-Rover. This was probably why the half-shaft snapped as I jerkily drove the vehicle out of the Sharland's drive, providing an anti-climax to our send-off. However the local agents replaced it immediately and also offered me a practical tip when driving the heavily-laden vehicle – always start in low ratio, four-wheel drive – make the first gear change into high ratio. This advice got us well into the desert before my clumsiness broke the half-shaft again. In mitigation, however, the half-shaft was a weakness in earlier models of the Forward Control Land Rover.

One does not enter the Sahara Desert suddenly. Through Zinder as far as Agadez, the well-graded sandy track meandered through vegetation which changed imperceptibly from Sudan Savanna to Sahel grassland. The scarce surface water soon became apparent when we saw herds of long-horned Zebu cattle congregated around the wells. By a system of ropes and pulleys, cattle or camels were used to draw the water up in huge cow-hide bags, which were emptied into the troughs.

We arrived in Agadez Saturday midday and were held up over the weekend. At the central administrative offices, attractively built of mud brick and cool inside with walls seemingly a yard thick, the authorities took our passports then closed till Monday, probably to ensure that we did not miss anything of the delights of Agadez. We used the time to check our vehicles and look round the large market, staying the two nights with a Spanish veterinary officer and his wife, who were delighted to put us up. Recruited for the JP15 rinderpest eradication scheme, they did not get many visitors. Fortunately he spoke a little English.

Collecting our passports on the Monday and in return passing over a couple of packets of Russian cigarettes – I knew we would find a use for them – we tackled the next stretch of our journey, undoubtedly the worst. Our routine by this time was to have a break of a few hours –

a siesta – during the hottest part of the day. We tried to avoid driving more than 200 miles a day. Night driving was out of the question because of the danger of losing the way.

From Agadez we headed towards the southern Algerian border-post at In Guezzam, following the mass of tracks in the otherwise featureless sandy desert. The withered grasses soon gave way to pebbly desert and then there was no vegetation whatsoever. The dark patches of stony gravel provided an excellent surface on which to drive, but the Sansoms had to be wary of the light-coloured patches of soft sand. We pulled them through one patch, and found that our vehicle, with the larger wheels, lower ratio gear-box and higher clearance had little trouble getting through.

Late afternoon, faced with a patch of badly churned-up soft sand just short of In Guezzam, we camped for the night. One of Peter's gems of advice had been that soft sand was always much firmer in the early morning. At dawn the next day we arrived at the little outpost of In Guezzam, where the mud-built buildings of the army post were shaded by a few tamarisk trees through which the wind sighed. Their well had a green scum on the surface of the water, so we declined their offer to fill up as we had plenty of water.

In these former French territories, I was able to converse in a sort of schoolboy French with the indigenous officials we encountered. Their French was precise, not heavily accented, idiom-free, and readily understood, that is by me, though June achieved more with a beaming smile. The Algerians spoke French much in the same way that Nigerians spoke English.

The young Algerian Commandant and one of his soldiers decided to accompany us to Tamanrasset, one in each vehicle. Whereas the Sansom's Land Rover had a bench seat in front, ours only had the hot engine cover between driver and passenger, so the Commandant reclined in the back on our bedding roll, seemingly very comfortable, though communication was almost impossible. Their help and guidance were of great value, even though they forced the pace a bit, ever worried about sandstorms which were notoriously bad on this stretch. I am sure they were also looking forward to the flesh-pots of Tamanrasset. We guessed that they intended to have a few days local leave there.

The slower speed of our Land Rover was a handicap on this stretch. I got little respite through a day that seemed endless and drove virtually for hours. Every time I caught up with the swifter vehicle, away they would go again. We followed a profusion of lorry tracks along what appeared to be several wide dry ancient river beds. Our guides showed us several short-cuts, which seemed to cut corners across virgin sand. We were entirely in their hands, but they knew what they were doing.

Late that same afternoon, having driven over 200 miles almost nonstop, I called a halt some fifty miles short of Tamanrasset. Even hot sweet refreshing mint tea brewed up on the spot, would not persuade me from my avowed intention of spending the night there. I was physically all-in and told them so in my best barrackroom Hindustani.

By this time we were into the foothills, if that be the correct term, of the Ahaggar Mountains, a huge volcanic massif in southern Algeria more or less in the centre of the Sahara. Eroded pyramids of basalt boulders or flat-topped hills and small patches of desert grass, like spinifex, appeared along the side of the track. We finally reached Tamanrasset, at an altitude of over 4,000 feet, early the next morning along a well-graded track that steadily climbed upwards. We pulled in behind the hotel amongst a grove of tamarisk trees.

Here we had our first taste of petty officialdom. A group of Algerian gendarmes arrived, and one walked around the vehicle. In front of our vehicle's radiator grill I had placed our table marker from the last Caledonian Ball we had attended the previous November. On the metal plaque was the St Andrew's Cross and beneath it our name in large letters. The gendarmes became quite agitated and it took me some time to realise that they thought we were supporters of Rhodesia's Ian Smith, who had declared U. D. I. only a few months previously. With great diplomacy I removed the offending plaque and later bought the gendarmes a beer in the hotel.

Scattered throughout the mountainous areas of the Sahara Desert are pools or watercourses of permanent water called *Gueltas*, generally lying along geological faults, or where basalt has flowed over older rocks. One we were shown, *Guelta Afilale*, several miles from Tamanrasset lay at an altitude of nearly 7,000 feet and looked so delightful that we decided to camp there for a few days to do a spot of serious bird study. Cautiously driving the vehicle across a bumpy kilometre of basalt boulders, we camped on the bank of this *Guelta* and within a short time had the narrow strip of greenery festooned with mist-nets, many of them suspended at a height across the *Guelta* on wires secured to rocks at the sides. Perhaps as well, because on our first night the braying of semi-wild donkeys kept us awake and they had as much right to the water as we did.

The many birds in the *Guelta* were no doubt attracted by the water, vegetation and abundant insects. Amongst the local species were several I could not identify, even when caught in the nets and handled. I skinned and preserved a selection of them for the British Museum and made notes of their description, calls and behaviour.

The weak but musical trumpet-like calls of trumpeter bullfinches, with their pastel pink head, breast and back, were heard throughout the day. A white-rumped black-chat had tucked its nest, containing three young, behind a rock on the bank. Pale crag martins sipped water on the wing gliding across the rock pools, as did migrant martins and swallows. Sandgrouse arrived noisily early or late in the day, wading into the water before drinking to wet their underparts. This adaptation to desert living allowed them to carry water back to their young out in the dry barren desert. We sampled a couple of the plentiful Rock doves to relieve the monotony of our diet of dried and tinned foods.

We caught several species of palearctic migrants, mainly yellow wagtails and swallows, though other familiar friends like nightingales, garden and willow warblers, tree pipits and woodchat shrikes also dropped in. Others seen but not netted were whinchats, redstarts, red-throated pipits and wheatears. They seemed to drop in just because they were overflying a favourable feeding area. The few weights of yellow wagtails which I obtained suggested that they still had adequate reserves to continue further.

One morning when the sun had warmed the rocks a little, we watched some white storks circling on the thermals until almost out of sight, whereupon they then drifted northwards on the light wind. Our only reminder of civilisation, the unmistakable silhouette of a Nigeria-bound VC10 with its two pairs of engines mounted at the rear, passed over so high that we required binoculars to see it.

In addition to semi-wild donkeys, we saw several feral camels, one of which walked sedately along the watercourse ducking under every net I had raised on wires, how fortunate I had them raised high. Gazelle, jackals, hares, even bats, came to water. Quaint little creatures like guinea pigs honeycombed the banks with their burrows. Later we learnt they were called *Gundis*. From this animal the parasite *Toxoplasma gondi* was first-isolated.

Idyllic as the place was, we had to move on after about ten days, visiting the Hermitage at Assekrem on our way back to Tamanrasset. The Hermitage at over 9,000 feet perpetuated the memory of Père de Foucault who worked amongst the Touaregs and was assassinated by rival tribesmen during the Great War. French monks looked after the small stone-built museum and chapel and maintained a weather station there. Dependent for their water on what rain they caught, huge cisterns had been excavated by hand in the basalt rock. The view from the top was stupendous. Rugged volcanic peaks and fluted basaltic cones stretched in all directions as far as the eye could see.

We stayed two nights in the hotel at Tamanrasset to freshen up a bit as the water at the *Guelta* had been icy-cold. After completing lengthy formalities we headed north on a well-graded but dreadfully corrugated track across the Tropic of Capricorn, around the French atomic base at In Eker and down the Arak Gorges to the foot of the escarpment. Some twenty miles further we filled all our water containers from a spring at Tadjemout and this was the last good water we found, as from here onwards the water seemed to get increasingly brackish.

Crossing the Plain of Tidikelt between In Salah and Reggane, we followed a line of oil drums spaced at half kilometre intervals across otherwise flat featureless sandy desert on a dreadfully corrugated track with stifling heat in the high forties Celsius. On this stretch a spring in the carburettor broke and the engine started racing, I messed up a gear change and snap went the half-shaft. We continued to an oasis called Aoulef on the front wheel drive and were delighted to find a small detachment of French Foreign Legion there. Equally delighted to see us, they made us welcome, even providing an Arab mechanic to replace the half-shaft, while I stood beside him checking the workshop manual.

During our two days in Aoulef, we were entertained regally. A Dutch student showed us neolithic implements and an old *Fougara* – an underground tunnel system which had brought water to Aoulef from the mountains to the south. Vertical shafts were sunk at regular intervals and connected beneath the surface, so the line of the system was shown by the piles of excavated material beside each shaft. Much of the old tunnel had collapsed. We were shown fossilised trees nearby, and in the irrigated patches in the oasis itself we saw several migrant wagtails and pipits, but did not bother to try and net them.

Along the sandy track past Reggane to Adrar, birds were plentiful. Bifasciated larks, known also as hoopoe larks, were nondescript brownish birds showing a flash of white on the wings as they flew up in front of the vehicle, just like miniature hoopoes. Coursers and wheatears were also conspicuous. Frequently swallows flew low in front of the vehicle. We skirted the Great Western Sand Sea on a proper road and reached Beni Abbes on the 21st April, nearly a month after we left Kano.

Beni Abbes, an important regional centre, enchanted us. Here we met André Dupuy from the Museum in Paris, netting migrant birds after they had accomplished the greater part of their journey. He was in the Research Centre, an admirable institution set up for scientists studying desert ecology and other aspects of the Sahara Desert.

With a back-drop of the enormous dunes of the Sand Sea and a fort, the Centre nestled on the slopes of a wadi and consisted of a Laboratory, a Museum full of neolithic implements and mineral specimens, a small botanical garden showing the few desert plants and a zoo containing desert animals, including a cheetah and a small colony of endearing *Gundi* whose acquaintance we had already made at the *Guelta*. One glass-fronted box appeared to contain only sand, but after dark by torchlight we found several horned vipers, which showed their displeasure at the torchlight by an awesome rasping sound as they reburied themselves in the sand.

The wide window of the laboratory faced down the dry water course to the date *Palmerie* in the distance, where Dupuy had several mist-nets. Any birds caught were brought up to the laboratory by his retinue of staff. This was bird-netting *par excellence*. June and I spent a day shaking the dust of the desert out of everything, then Dupuy took us out to a rapidly drying salt lake, *Chott Daiet Tiour*, about 150 miles from Beni Abbes, where we spent a week in solitude but for the myriads of migrant birds that streamed in from the south.

Mist-nets soon festooned the sparse vegetation along one side and we caught many migrant passerines and waders. Dupuy kept us fully occupied also chasing, and banding, several hundred flightless Ruddy Shelduck ducklings across acres of thick tenacious mud, for by this time the lake was rapidly drying up. We dined well, for André's cook performed wonders with those few unfortunate ducklings which broke their legs in their mad scrambles to get away from us. Dupuy had less English than I had French, but we had a common language in Latin when discussing bird species. Some acquaintance of his had taught him the chorus from the Hippopotamus song, and we were entertained by 'Mud, mud, glorious mud . . .' sung by him with great gusto in an outrageous accent.

Returning to Beni Abbes for a further five nights, we revelled in the luxury of the accommodation provided at the Centre. For a pittance we had a nice clean room, abundant hot water, and all meals thrown in. This included Pernod aperitifs before we dined and cheap but very palatable Algerian rosé wines with the meals.

Saddened that it all had to end, we still had ten days driving in front of us and were impatient to get back to England to see Roger and the family and finalise arrangements for Australia. At Tamanrasset I had called at the post office and found a letter from my mother. In it I was delighted to find the firm offer of a job in Perth, Western Australia.

Our route northwards, aiming for the Straits of Gibraltar, lay through

Morocco, but the border crossing at Colomb Bechar quite near Beni Abbes was closed. Instead we headed for a small border post at Figuig where, after the usual interminable formalities, we wended our way along a narrow track through a no-man's land festooned with barbed-wire and also past a minefield on either side, which the Automobile Association in Britain had already warned us about, because the Moroccans and Algerians were almost at war.

We were received cordially on the Moroccan side and with a general feeling of well-being and eager to make up lost time I broke one of my cardinal rules and drove on after dark. In the desert, driving in the dark was inadvisable because of the danger of losing the track, but here we were on a well-graded gravel track that allowed us to travel fast.

Several dry sandy river beds were crossed on concrete causeways, dipping down, across and up the other side. With far too much confidence I went over a couple at speed. The third one nearly proved our undoing. As the vehicle dipped down and the headlights illuminated the causeway, I was horrified to see a gaping hole big enough to take quite comfortably everything we had to offer, Land Rover and all. I skidded to a halt, almost teetering on the brink of this dreadful abyss, then hastily backed up because much of the causeway still standing was eroded by flood waters. These watercourses flowed from the high Atlas Mountains southwards into the desert and we learnt later that serious flooding had occurred when the snows melted earlier. Again I heeded one of Peter Woods' gems, that many people get drowned in the desert.

Crossing that particular dry river bed higher up and proceeding on our way much more cautiously for another hour, we were astonished at the amount of wild-life we saw. Little hopping mice, I think they were gerbils, were everywhere. In the headlights we got a good view of a Fennec, the desert fox, chasing the gerbils, making short pounces, its huge bat-like ears pricked forward. We eventually pulled off the road and bedded down.

The next three days in Morocco were delightful. From the market town of Ksar Es Souk we motored up the Gorges du Ziz and over the

High Atlas Mountains to Midelt where snow was visible not far from the hotel where we spent the night. The air sparkled like champagne and over the Col du Zad there were cedars and a profusion of small alpine plants. At Fez we decided no more discomfort for us in the cramped back of the Land Rover. We felt we had earned a night in the Grand Hotel and a young Moroccan lad gave us a superb tour of the market that evening.

Although aiming for the Straits of Gibraltar, I somehow anticipated seeing the Mediterranean first, into which we might have dashed fully clothed. Alas, we first saw a cold, rough Atlantic Ocean south of Tangier. Crossing to Algeciras in southern Spain after a night in Tangier, we finally arrived back in England on the 17th May.

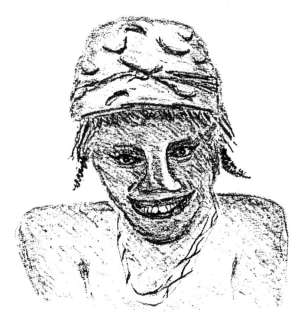

Fulani maiden – "*Sannu Bature*"

At Stonehenge in the Salisbury Plains near Roger's school, we had a little ceremony to celebrate our return to Britain. Carried with us as part of our precious emergency water reserve, was a twelve gallon container of Vom water which we had not used. We thought it fitting that we should carefully decant this memento from Nigeria around the perimeter fence at Stonehenge.

Vom revisited in 1974

NOT LONG AFTER WE DEPARTED FROM NIGERIA, driving out through Daura on its northern border, the backlash against the Ibos in the north resulted in the massacre of countless thousands of them, many on the Plateau. Their declaration of independence with the formation of their own State, Biafra, and the tragic Biafran War – The Brother's War – deeply scarred the country. Those Ibos not killed fled the north back to their homelands. We were glad to learn later from expatriate friends that some Ibos we had known in Vom had survived, particularly those who had sensibly run for their lives before the main bloodshed started. Emmanuel Ezebuiro, Acting Director when I left, had several narrow escapes getting away and he never returned to the Directorate.

In Vom essential services were badly affected and vaccine production ceased or was severely disrupted. I heard on the grapevine that vaccine seed material had got mixed up and strange mixtures were being issued. Several years later rinderpest swept over the borders of the country from the north-east, aided by the decreased vigilance of the field services and new generations of susceptible cattle, and caused a massive outbreak. In 1966 the incidence of rinderpest in Nigeria had dropped almost to zero as a result of JP15, but pockets of infection survived in territories further east, especially in those countries which were torn apart by civil unrest.

Well settled into a new job in Australia, I returned to Nigeria for a short visit with my family in January 1974. The effects of a seven year drought in the Sahel were very apparent even at Kano Airport. We spent a few days in the Catering Rest House at Vom, meeting there Forrest Laing, whom I had seen in Maiduguri on our trip to the Waza Game Reserve in the French Cameroons over ten years previously and on a few occasions since. He was in Vom on an O.D.A. appointment.

A Senegal Hoopoe was feeding nestlings behind our chalet, where else but in a nest below ground in a broken-down septic tank. I was told later that the Catering Rest House had been an important military installation during the war for dispensing troop comforts, a brothel, no less.

Jide Shonekan was Acting Director and looked after us well, providing us with transport to Jos so that we could call on old friends there. We found a Danish couple, Freddy and Kirsten Lund, still in their house there. Freddy had been the Provincial Veterinary Officer in Jos for many years.

Dantiyi and Badung visited us at the C. R. H. and looked well. Both seemed to have invested wisely the gratuities I had given them. Soon after we had left Vom in 1966, I received a letter of thanks from Dantiyi's elder brother, Davou, explaining that he could not have completed his nurse's training at Vom Mission without the money we had paid Dantiyi.

I was delighted to see my old friend from Lagos days, James Adeleye, on the staff at the Farm, and he greeted me with obvious pleasure. In the Laboratory, Johnson Onovo had only just returned from the south, having fled during the massacres. Never one to smile much, he seemed to have even less to smile about, but we had a chat about the good old times. Jonah was still there, as were Nayaba Vom and Sale, who both eyed me as if I had returned from the grave to claim some long-unpaid loan.

There were many new faces amongst the professional staff, some with qualifications from Russia or Central Europe behind the Iron Curtain, but no one I spoke to seemed to have much idea of what he was doing. Broken equipment littered the rooms and the verandahs at the back of the buildings. Still hanging on the wall of my old office was a dusty item of equipment for producing distilled water, which had broken just before I left and never had been repaired.

Our former house in Vom had another residence built in the front

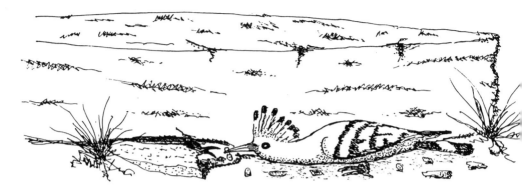

Hoopoe at nest

garden and both looked a trifle unkempt. As we drove slowly past I wondered, '. . . And what of the wagtails?'

Hilary Fry had earlier told me he had a post-graduate zoology student from Aberdeen working in Vom. Brian Wood was studying for his PhD on the wagtails in the same roost in the same patch of sugar cane and he took us out netting one evening. His technique was much the same as ours. I was interested to learn that by 1974, many recoveries had been reported, and his findings substantially supported the results Dave Ebbutt and I had published in a brief communication nearly ten years previously.

How gratifying that at least some of my work had been of value.

Acronyms & Abbreviations

ATMN	Amalgamated Tin Mines of Nigeria.
BG	*Bayan Gida* (Hausa), – 'Behind the house' – Latrine.
BOAC	British Overseas Airways Corporation.
BOU	British Ornithologist's Union.
BTO	British Trust for Ornithology
CSIRO	Commonwealth Scientific & Industrial Research Organisation.
DGV	Dried Goat Virus (a vaccine against Rinderpest).
EEC	European Economic Community.
EPU	Egg Production Unit.
FAO	Food & Agricultural Organisation.
FDVR	Federal Department of Veterinary Research.
FMD	Foot & Mouth Disease.
FPV	Fowl Pox Vaccine.
IBR	Infectious Bovine Rhinotracheitis.
JP15	Joint Project 15 (an internationally-funded campaign against Rinderpest).
LIC	Livestock Investigation Centre.
LRV	Lapinised Rinderpest Vaccine.
LSCS	Lump Sum Compensation Scheme ('Lumpers').
MOD	Ministry for Overseas Development.
NDV	Newcastle Disease Vaccine.
NESCO	Nigerian Electricity Supply Company.

NITR	Nigerian Institute for Trypanosomiasis Research.
NPC	Northern People's Congress.
OCS	Overseas Civil Service.
ODA	Overseas Development Authority.
PPR	*Peste des petits ruminants* – a Rinderpest-like disease of sheep and goats described by French workers in West Africa.
PWD	Public Works Department.
TC	Tissue Culture.
TCRV	Tissue-cultured Rinderpest Vaccine.
UDI	Unilateral Declaration of Independence.
USAID	United States Aid.
WACMR	West African Council for Medical Research.
WAITR	West African Institute for Trypanosomiasis Research.